Eat Well with Nell

Eat Well with Nell

Food to Make You Feel Good

Nell Nelson

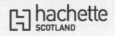
hachette
SCOTLAND

First published in 2009 by
HACHETTE SCOTLAND, an imprint of
Hachette UK

1

Cataloguing in Publication Data is available from the British Library

ISBN 978 0 7553 1855 1

Designed by Ben Cracknell
Typeset in Bell MT by Avon DataSet Ltd,
Bidford on Avon, Warwickshire

Printed and bound in Great Britain by
Clays Ltd, St Ives plc

Hachette Scotland's policy is to use papers that are natural, renewable and
recyclable products and made from wood grown in sustainable forests. The
logging and manufacturing processes are expected to conform to the
environmental regulations of the country of origin.

Hachette Scotland
An Hachette UK Company
338 Euston Road
London NW1 3BH

www.hachettescotland.co.uk
www.hachette.co.uk

Contents

Introduction

Food Writing, Television Presenting and Nutrition

I love food, and everything associated with food: foraging in shops, farmers' markets and supermarkets, reading recipe books, cooking, writing, talking and tasting food, and of course eating. So on reflection, my stomach has definitely influenced the path of my life.

I remember when I was seven, entering swimming competitions at the local outdoor pool; not for the joy of winning or having my name in the newspaper, but for the greedy delight in winning a whole box of chocolates. I was very lucky and my parents loved food; they encouraged my brother and me to cook. I've found menu plans written in my ten-year-old hand for dinner parties using a mix of Delia Smith's original 1970s *How to Cheat at Cooking* and *The World's Best Soufflés*. The only way I can explain the subsequent

2 · **Eat Well with Nell**

diversity and range of my cooking, is that these two cookbooks must both have been on the lowest accessible bookshelf.

As long as I can remember I have kept a diary in which I have recorded every day what I ate, not as some kind of food diary which I now ask my clients to keep – to help them work out whether they have any allergies – but as a trigger to remind me of events. 'Strawberry mousse for school dinner today ' takes me back to being eleven years old, sitting at a long trestle table in sheer heaven with a huge bowl of synthetic pink e numbers in front of me.

At university I joined the Arabic Society, not to discover more about the Seven Pillars of Islam but to be a member of its supper club, make gorgeous Middle Eastern dishes and experiment with sesame seeds, rosewater, tahini and gallons of olive oil, ingredients which our student flat kitty wasn't up to subsidising.

Attracted by the bright lights and long lunches of advertising, I went to London to work as a copywriter, dreaming up ads for Mercedes trucks and jelly babies. To liven up a long and cold London winter, I took Afro-Caribbean cooking evening classes. Every week we would arrive with our shopping list of exotica: bags of chopped up goat, large green unwieldy plantains and even a bottle of rum. I learned to make a mean goat curry and mix a strong rum punch. Based on my newly acquired knowledge of the cuisine, I became a restaurant reviewer for the Afro-Caribbean section of *Time Out London Eating and Drinking Guide*. I cycled all over London and during that time must have eaten a flock of goat, fields of rice and beans, washed down with copious amounts of rum punch.

The Lure of the East

A friend was working in Hong Kong as a journalist and said 'come out for a holiday'. I did and loved it – and stayed for ten years. In Hong Kong, being a reviewer of Afro-Caribbean food was not the most obvious credential for writing about Asian food, but I had business cards printed with 'Nell Nelson, Food and Travel Writer' and launched myself into the Hong Kong food world. I had been told about the 'Hong Kong handshake' where, in any social situation before a 'hello, pleased to meet you' is even uttered, a name card is thrust towards you with both hands. At restaurant press parties, I would present people with a newly minted Nell Nelson business card and they would look at my job title of food and travel writer and say, 'I would love to do that' and I would mutter under my breath 'So would I.'

When the supportive food editor on Hong Kong's English language newspaper *The South China Morning Post* gave me a break and asked me to write a food review of a new Ethiopian restaurant, I was off, with a keen appetite and large notebook. For the next ten years I ate for Hong Kong; I wrote food articles in which my mission was to discover the ten best carrot cakes, dim sum, Singapore Slings etc. in the Territory. Invariably I left my research to the last moment and ended up eating ten baskets of barbecued pork buns or drinking pints of bright red Slings three hours before deadline. I also took a Young Women's Christian Association (YWCA) course in dim sum making and made the largest prawn dumplings my Cantonese classmates had ever seen, prompting them to say to me, using typical Cantonese directness,

'If you opened a restaurant, it would go out of business.'

I then found myself editing the glossy food magazine *Asian Home Gourmet* and I loved commissioning and organising gorgeous food shoots; and eating the props. I also wrote a weekly column for *The South China Morning Post* called Nosh which was my public food diary, and my licence to roam and eat. The column expanded to include recipes which I then included in a book called *Eat Cook Hong Kong* which was based on what I had in fact done – eaten, then found out the recipes and learned how to cook them.

Hong Kong is also a wonderful base for cycling around Asia and, over the years, eating and pedalling complemented each other perfectly. I thought 'I've cracked it; I can eat as much as I like and not get fat.' And indeed I had.

Travelling on Two Wheels

I first cycled from Hong Kong to Hanoi in Vietnam and discovered the joy of choosing my own vegetables for a bespoke stir-fry on a Guangzhou back street and the time of day when fresh spring roll sellers hit the Vietnamese streets to roll unruly beansprouts, minced pork and tiny freshwater shrimps into tight transparent bundles. A harder pedal was the one we did from China to Pakistan on the Karakoram Highway across the Kunjerab Pass on rough roads ravaged by avalanches with a backdrop of snow-topped mountains. I ate lamb and cumin kebabs cooked over hot coals on massive metal skewers, and apricots dried by the hot Hunza valley sun. In Myanmar I discovered a caffeine-hit salad made with fermented green tea leaves, fresh soya bean snacks, and learned that the British tradition of tea and cakes at 4pm is still part of the everyday culture.

After ten years, like some kind of giant locust, I had eaten and cycled my way through most of Asia and I was ready to leave Hong Kong for grazing on pastures new. I had been to

Australia and had been struck by the quality and variety of the food available. Thanks to strict laws on importing food, immigrants from all over the world had learned to grow and produce their favourite ingredients on the rich Australian soil – olive oil, wine, cheeses etc. – and so I decided to cycle to this food Mecca and collect recipes along the way for a cookbook which I would call *Out of the Wok onto the Barbie.* I intended to cycle on my own from Hong Kong to Australia, through Vietnam, Cambodia, Thailand, Malaysia, Singapore, across the Indonesian archipelago, then down the east coast of Australia from Cairns to Sydney.

The whole trip affirmed my love of eating, cycling, meeting people and writing. I wrote a weekly food column for *The South China Morning Post* with restaurant tips on the various capitals of south-east Asia I cycled through. I filed my copy from hot, fan-whirred internet cafes; sipped fresh orange juice and coffee sweetened with condensed milk; took readers from Vietnamese French colonial shuttered restaurants which served elegant crème brûlée, to cocktails at the Phnom Penh Foreign Correspondents Club; introduced them to a sophisticated watermelon, basil and feta salad in an über-cool Bangkok bar to Singapore Slings and chicken satays under palm trees in the Lion City. I wrote of Balinese spicy fruit salads which simultaneously bring tears of pain and pleasure; of the joy of discovering creamy egg Portuguese egg tarts in Dili, East Timor; of the long straight sugar-cane and banana palm-lined of roads of Queensland, Australia; of the promise of huge steaks which overhang the plate, and of banana bread and jam from the banana plantations of Australia.

It wasn't all easy. Severe Acute Respiratory Syndrome (SARS) broke out just before I left, so while there was never any trouble finding a room for the night, it meant there were few travellers to meet. I did meet some cyclists – usually going in the opposite direction. People were extraordinarily friendly to me, and a bicycle is a real leveller; in Asia everyone cycles. Children go to school, three on a bike; women cycle to work with long gloves on their arms to protect themselves from the sun and farmers cycle to market with pigs strapped over the back wheel. I learned a little of each language, and the first word was 'delicious'. 'Delicious' is the best opening line in the world. Forget 'Where's the toilet?' 'Two beers please' or 'Do you have a light?' 'Delicious' doesn't just open oven doors it opens all doors, and I met lots of people and tasted amazing market foods that I might not have done.

I caught a cold in Vietnam after getting soaked in the monsoon rain and couldn't get dry again. Then I got food poisoning in West Timor, Indonesia and it was while recovering that, for the first time in my life, it dawned on me that food is necessary to live on, but not in a Bridget Jones-like way to be monitored and agonised over. No, now I needed food as fuel, and the only way out of Kefa, a remote mountain village to which I had cycled, was on my bicycle. The public transport I had seen on the twisting well-tarmaced road to Kefa consisted of tiny blue minibuses packed full of people, chickens and sacks of rice; I had even seen a live cow covered with banana leaves on the roof of a bus! Just the thought of an over-packed, over-heated bus with live chickens and clove-scented cigarettes made me nauseous. I remember ransacking my brain trying to think which foods had given me the most energy. I had never run out of 'steam' while eating the south-east Asian diet which is naturally very healthy – lots of carbohydrates; rice and noodles, vegetables, and a little meat and fruit, together with sweet treats such as banana fritters for instant energy, when faced by a hill – so I forced myself to eat bony fish, rice and bananas.

Also, I have to admit, retail therapy can never be ignored in times of hardship and lack of food. There were few shops in Timor, but on my way to Dili I stopped by a small stall selling woven sarongs. I bought a small pretty orange and red strip of material and the pleasure was so great, I instantly felt better. I still have it and it makes me smile.

Seven months, nine countries, five thousand miles and five punctures later, I arrived in Sydney. I had planned to look for food-writing work in Sydney as I was attracted by Sydney-siders' totally international yet very Australian food culture, but while cycling in New South Wales I had one of those moments where a life-changing thought suddenly hits you, and mine was about food. I had been cycling for about four hours in the morning and was ready for my morning break. There were few places to stop on this remote stretch of road and I spotted a caravan park which had a café. There were two choices of cake: Rocky Road, a marshmallow, nut and chocolate confection, or Millionaire toffee shortbread – a great Scottish staple – which my mother makes. While weighing up Rocky Road against toffee shortbread I had a blinding flash: I'd have the toffee shortbread, and I would end my journey in Sydney and fly back to Scotland – to the 'land of toffee shortbread'.

Home So Sweet Home

My cycling trip made a huge impact on my life in so many ways. I would recommend anyone to take the plunge and follow their dream, not just for the anticipation, pleasure and satisfaction from doing what you have always wanted to do, but for the positive knock-on effects. After having experienced the importance of food in relationship to physical exercise and mood, I wanted to learn more about how food affects all our actions. So I studied for a Diploma in Nutritional Therapy with the College of Naturopathic Medicine, which has a college in Edinburgh.

Meanwhile, I had been so impressed by the passion people in Asia had for their food, and their pride in locally produced ingredients, that I hoped my own country might too have a similarly rich seam. While cycling in Bali a friend studying at Sydney film school had flown out to meet me, and we had made a seven-minute film of me tracking down the recipe for fish baked in banana leaves which we called *The Woman Who Ate Asia*. I wrote a proposal for a television programme called *The Woman Who Ate Scotland* in which I proposed to cycle and eat my way round Scotland. I sent my proposal off to production company Tern Television with my promo video from Bali. I was incredibly lucky; STV were looking for a food travel programme and they liked the idea and said yes, 'start filming now' – in darkest December in Scotland. Clad in Gore-Tex from head to toe, cycling up and down the same deep snow track shouting through the snowflakes to a moving camera was a far cry from weaving down brilliant green paddy field-lined roads in flip-flops, but I loved making the series and learning more about the local produce from traditional Arbroath Smokies to the latest Scottish crop, garlic.

We made an eight-part series of *The Woman Who Ate Scotland* for STV in which I cycled and ate all over Scotland from Edinburgh to Inverness. The most exciting discovery was the realisation that my own country has an incredible history, is the source of wonderful foods and also contains people who are passionate about food. Some of them and their recipes are featured in this book. The first series of *The Woman*

Who Ate Scotland was well received and another eight-part series was commissioned which took me from New Zealand bakers in Glasgow to the remote north-west coast of Scotland; from the joys of preparing and eating salmon sushi by the sea, to Shetland for seaweed-fed lamb. Even after making sixteen programmes, there is still so much more of Scotland left to eat and cycle.

It's Not All Mung Beans and Wheatgrass

After graduating with a diploma in Nutritional Therapy I started working as a nutritionist with Neal's Yard Remedies in Edinburgh, and through my practice have learned so much more about nutrition and about helping people eat better. You know you need to eat more vegetables, oily fish and wholegrains, but the hard thing is knowing how to – clients need inspiring recipes such as sweet potato and coconut soup or trout stuffed with pearl barley, dates and ginger. Creating personalised recipe books for my clients sparked off the idea for this book, *Eat Well with Nell.*

Mung beans and wheatgrass have their place – I do like mung beans, though I feel wheatgrass is an acquired taste – but this book is about discovering the pleasure and enjoyment of healthy eating. This book is for anyone who wants a pointer towards eating their way to good health, but it is not meant to be so hard-core healthy that you buy the book, use it for a week, find it too antisocial and hard to stick to, and pack it straight off to Oxfam. The recipes are designed to inspire you to cook and to enjoy eating – there is sugar, there is chocolate, there is cheese, even wine, but enjoy them in moderation. If you have serious health concerns, then it is worth seeking specialist advice from a nutritionist or doctor.

But I don't want you to eat something just because it is good for you – eat it because it is delicious – in whatever language.

My Mission

My big cycle trip was the start of many journeys – physically through nine countries – but it also sparked a major food discovery: that food is for life, yes, but for a better life. Of course it should taste good and be a means of cementing friendships, but also it can enhance your life – offering you boundless energy, good health, the weight you want to be, restful sleep, good skin, hair, strong bones and a happy outlook. This is the journey I want to take you on – don't worry, I won't suggest you cycle a hundred miles a day. I simply hope I can make you feel the best you have ever felt and encourage you to learn to love food as your friend, and take life on and love it – so start now and read on to find out how.

> But I don't want you to eat something just because it is good for you — eat it because it is delicious — in whatever language

Book Tools

This is the key to eating well – if you read nothing else, read this:

Blood Sugar Balance

Balancing the amount of sugar or glucose in your blood is the key to good health and the principal message of *Eat Well with Nell*. Get this right and the rest will follow – in fact the remainder of the book is basically all about helping you fine-tune this simple advice:

Make sure you have a balanced level of sugar in your blood at all times and you will have limitless energy, concentration and enthusiasm for life.

The main source of energy is carbohydrate; your body can use protein and fat for energy, but it takes a lot longer for the body to digest and release their energy, so it prefers carbs. Carbohydrates are broken down into glucose which your body can use and store for energy. The best way to manage your blood sugar is to eat small and regular amounts of a mixture of complex carbohydrates, which means it takes longer for the carbohydrates in your food to get broken down into glucose which is then released into your bloodstream gradually.

Glycemic Index and Load

This blood sugar process has been turned into a science and you may have read about it as the Glycemic Index (GI). The GI is a numerical scale which measures the rate at which carbohydrate in food is broken down in the digestive tract and the rate that sugars are absorbed into the bloodstream, on a scale from 1 to 100. Foods that release their sugars more slowly have fewer points than those that are released quickly. Here is a table listing the GI of some of the most common carbohydrate foods.

High GI Foods (GI 60–100)

Food	GI
Baguette	95
Banana	65
Beetroot (cooked)	64
Cantaloupe melon	65
Couscous (cooked)	65
Chocolate chip muffin	65
Jelly beans	80
Mars Bar	68
Parsnips (boiled)	97
Pineapple	66
Potatoes (cooked)	70
Raisins	64

Pumpkin	75
Rice cakes	82
Watermelon	72

Medium GI Foods (40–59)

Food	GI
Banana cake	47
Basmati rice	58
Buckwheat (cooked)	40
Brown rice (not quick cook)	50
Bulghur wheat (cooked)	48
Carrots (cooked)	49
Chickpeas (canned)	42
Digestive biscuit	59
Kidney beans (tinned)	52
Mango	55
Muesli	56
Peas	48
Porridge (cooked with water)	42
Orange	44
Sweetcorn (canned)	55
Sourdough rye bread	55
Spaghetti (white cooked)	41
Sweet potatoes	54

Low GI Foods (1–39)

Food	GI
Apple	38
Apricots (dried)	31
Cherries	22
Lentils (cooked)	30

Pear	38
Pearl barley (boiled)	25
Peanuts	14
Vegetables: asparagus, aubergine, cauliflower, tomato, greens	10
Yoghurt (low fat)	33
Spaghetti (wholewheat)	37
Soya beans	18

Figures courtesy of the University of Sydney, please see their website http://www.glycemicindex.com/ for more details.

You'll see that there are some anomalies in the GI tables – pineapples, parsnips and watermelon are in the high GI food category because they are high in easily accessed sugar, but they have other health benefits, so you can't compare a slice of watermelon to a Mars Bar. Cooking vegetables such as carrots raises their GI. Cooking allows the sugar to be released more quickly into the body so raw foods tend to have a lower GI. Cooking, however, while raising the GI also sometimes raises the uptake of vital antioxidants, so don't get too hung up with this table.

High GI foods tend to be the foods that people reach for when they need a quick energy fix, so not surprisingly muffins, along with chocolate chip muffins, baguettes and Mars Bars are all high GI foods (61–100) as they are quickly broken down to sugar.

Medium GI foods (40–59) are foods with a bit more 'bite' to them, i.e. it takes your body longer to break them down into sugar. They include foods such as rye bread, brown rice, sweet potato and wholewheat pasta, and some fruits such as oranges and mango.

Low GI foods (1–39) comprise the majority of vegetables, except for very sweet ones like carrots, peas and potatoes, so enjoy them as part of a meal. These can all be eaten more freely: artichokes, asparagus, aubergine, avocado, beetroot, broccoli, Brussels sprouts, bok choy, cauliflower, celeriac, celery, Chinese cabbage, courgette, onions, pepper, squash, tomato, turnip, watercress and yam. Leafy green vegetables are also good low GI foods: chicory, iceberg lettuce, kale, loose-leaf lettuce, mustard greens, rocket, sorrel, spinach and watercress. Some fruits such as pears and apples are low GI as are nuts, pulses and yoghurt. As long as you eat a balanced range of protein, good fats, complex carbohydrates and fruits and vegetables, it does not matter if they are low to middle GI.

Meat, fish and dairy have a more complicated structure of fat and protein, so they automatically fall into the low GI section as it takes your body longer to digest and release their energy.

Glycemic Load

You eat foods together so they are not isolated. Jumbo oats are good GI foods – you can almost see the fibres and endosperms etc. that will take time to be digested, but combine them with some raisins, which are a simple sugar, and 'heavens above' some golden syrup – which would normally go straight to the bloodstream – then you have a flapjack which is half good and half bad. The scientists add up the figures of the ingredients and divide to get an average and they call this the Glycemic Load (GL). You should be averaging a GL of around 80 per day, but most people's GL will be 120 and upwards.

But once you start involving tables, sums and scientists it gets complicated so it's not worth going too far down this route; it takes any fun out of food. But it is useful when it comes to blood sugar balance to try at all times to include a complex carbohydrate and protein, and some fibre and some unsaturated fat in any meal, so if you feel like a snack of say a raisin, have a few nuts (protein and fat) to slow down the speed at which the raisin's glucose content hits the bloodstream. Low GI foods tend to fill you up and keep you satisfied for longer, so you will feel less need to return to the stock of nuts and raisins.

Essential Food Groups

Carbohydrates

Some carbohydrates are better than others. Sugar or glucose comes from all the foods you eat – your body can turn carbohydrates, protein and fat into fuel, i.e. sugar – but the easiest source is from carbohydrates. All carbohydrate, which is the main source of energy for the body, gets broken down into sugar, but not all carbohydrates are equal. Even your epitome of dieting, a crispbread, will get broken down by the body into sugar, but the key to the whole blood sugar business is the speed with which the body breaks the food down into sugar. And the way to slow down the breakdown is by eating complex carbohydrate – i.e. foods which take the body longer to break down into sugar. These more complex carbohydrates are broken down into glucose slowly and stored as glycogen in the muscle cells and in the liver, until needed.

If glucose gradually enters your bloodstream, insulin levels will remain relatively constant to deal with this slow trickle. This means that glucose gradually enters the bloodstream, providing constant energy – sorry to make you sound like a battery, but that is quite a good analogy – so you won't suddenly feel tired, or faint, or crave a muffin, but enjoy longer lasting energy until eventually the glucose runs out and you need to stock up again. But it is a gradual descent – a green ski slope as opposed to the black killer run. Simple carbohydrates are easy for the body to break down too quickly into simple sugars. Naturally they're found in fruit and vegetables. Refined sugars are found in foods such as cakes, biscuits and pastries and some breakfast cereals. The more refined the carbohydrate, the faster the glucose is released into your blood.

Complex carbohydrates require more effort for the body to break down, so the glucose is released slowly. A good rule of thumb is that the more processed a food, the more likely that it will be broken down into sugar more quickly. Brown is good as brown means more of the grain has been left intact and is less processed. Examples of good slow-release carbohydrates are some of the more complex wholegrains which are readily available such as

- Brown rice
- Barley
- Oats
- Millet
- Spelt
- Rye
- Couscous
- Buckwheat and its pasta
- Wholewheat pasta
- Wholewheat pitta
- Oatcakes

You should be aiming for about six portions a day, spread throughout the day. A portion is quite small – 50g of uncooked grains or muesli, or one slice of wholemeal bread.

Proteins

Protein is the body's building and repair material. Protein in the form of amino acids is found in most foods, even vegetables. The body needs the amino acids it gets from animal and vegetable products to make protein. Meat and fish contain all eight essential amino acids.

It is best to opt for less saturated fat meats and also if possible to eat organic and free-range chicken, turkey and eggs. Organic free-range meat is thought to contain less saturated fat as the animals are able to exercise more, so are leaner and not artificially fattened up. Fish is also a good source of low-fat protein as are the vegetarian-friendly grain quinoa and soya products.

But there are also many more incredibly versatile protein choices which are often cheaper and carry greater health benefits. Pulses and legumes are a source of carbohydrate, but they also have some amino acids. Not as many as meat or fish, but if you combine a pulse such as chickpeas or beans with a grain such as rice, you can get all the essential amino acids your body needs to make protein. In many parts of the world where meat is scarce or the people subsist on a vegetarian diet, the combination of pulse and grain is a major source of protein – think of Mexican corn tortillas (grain) with refried beans (pulse) or an Indian chickpea curry with rice (pulse and grain). Indian stores tend to have a great range of pulses.

The body needs small and regular amounts of amino acids. If you consume excess amounts of protein, you make your body very acidic which is harmful to your tissues. Processing excess protein makes extra work for your body and what protein isn't needed will get stored as fat – ready to be broken down when the body needs it – so all those half-pound steaks are not turning into muscle but heading for the hips or other parts of the body with hungry fat-receptor cells.

The recommended amount of protein is two to three portions a day – about fifteen to twenty per cent of food on your plate should be proteins, and they should be quite easy to integrate. The Department of Health says the recommended daily intake of protein for adult men is 55.5g and 45g for women; 100g of chicken breast yields about 25g of protein so that is more than half a woman's quota.

Try to have a good variety in order to get a wide range of amino acids. Be wary of too much meat high in saturated fats.

One portion of protein is:

- A big spoonful of yoghurt with porridge
- A spread of nut butter on a piece of oatcake
- 100g serving of chicken or turkey
- 125g oily fish, white fish
- 2 eggs
- 3 tablespoons of nuts or seeds
- 4 tablespoons of cooked grains with 4 tablespoons pulses

Fats

The body loves fat – it harks back to the days when we were never sure where our next meal was coming from, so it was useful to be able to lay down fat for future use. Our body stores fat, whereas its first inclination with carbohydrates is to burn them, so if carbohydrate consumption is low, it may annoyingly decide to burn fewer calories (calories are the measure of fuel you need per day to live) during the day, rather than burn up the 'precious' supply of fat it has laid down.

Like everything in the food world there are good fats and bad fats. Good fats are the polyunsaturated fats found in nuts, seeds and oily fish; they contain omega 3 essential fatty acids which have myriad benefits. Bad fats are the saturated ones found in dairy products and meat, and should not be consumed to excess. The body does not like turning carbohydrates into body fat; it takes up more energy so it is not economic. It finds it easier therefore to turn fat to fat, as it can always make a home for more fat.

> The body loves fat

The recommended amount from the Department of Health is two to four portions of fat a day, and most of it should be unsaturated. This is pure fat, but lots of foods such as nuts, seeds, meat and dairy contain fat, so it's hard to isolate, but when it comes to pure fat, you don't need much. One portion is:

- 1 teaspoon butter
- 1 teaspoon cooking oil
- 1 tablespoon cream

Fibre

Fibre is wonderful as it slows down the speed at which sugar is absorbed into the bloodstream. It is found in most of the grain-based carbohydrates and all fruits and vegetables. For blood sugar management you should try to have some fibre with each meal. Fibre is also very good for maintaining a healthy intestine as it helps remove toxins and excess hormones from the body and speeds up the time it takes for food to pass through the body – you don't want digested food lingering in the intestines as it can ferment and the toxins and water get re-absorbed. Complex carbohydrates, as well as fruit and vegetables, especially with their skins, are all good sources of fibre.

These, together with nuts and seeds, all contribute to your fibre intake, so if you are taking the appropriate quantities of these you should be getting enough fibre. The Department of Health suggests 18g of fibre in food per day, but really you should be going for almost double that amount for good blood sugar management and a healthy bowel.

Good sources of insoluble and soluble fibre are:

- Pulses – beans and lentils and chickpeas
- Seeds and nuts
- Wholegrain foods such as wholewheat, spelt, buckwheat, millet, brown rice, barley, oats, rye
- Soybeans
- Fruit, especially with skin on like apples and pears
- Vegetables such as green beans, sweetcorn, cauliflower, celery and vegetables with skins like peas and broad beans

A 100g portion of muesli has 7.6g of fibre, whereas 100g of wholemeal bread (3 slices) has 8.1g and 100g of wholemeal pasta has 9g so you can see that if you go for lots of complex carbs and veggies you will easily consume more than the recommended minimum amount of fibre in a day without having to get out the scales.

Water

Your body is sixty to seventy per cent water, so it makes sense to ensure you are hydrated. Water is needed for every single bodily function. Just breathing uses up about 500ml a day, so try and make sure you are taking in about 1.5–2 litres a day. There is also water in food, so if you are eating lots of fruit and veggies, then your water levels should be quite high. If your urine is dark yellow, then you need to take in more water, until it becomes pale yellow.

Five-a-day

The Food Standards Agency is running a campaign called 'Five-a-day' which some food producers and supermarkets have embraced. It recommends you should eat five portions of fruit and vegetables a day. Fruit and vegetables should make up about a third of your daily diet. It is helpful to look at your diet to see if you are managing to meet this target, but I recommend you try for more than five portions, especially of vegetables. Fruit is quite high in sugar and could upset blood sugar balance, whereas vegetables – ideally green leafy and non-starchy – will if anything slow down blood sugar conversion due to their fibrous content, so perhaps you should try for three to four portions of fruit, and five portions or more of vegetables.

Here is a quick guide to the quantities and types of fruit and vegetables you should be aiming for in order to 'eat to feel well'. I have used cups as they are an easy measure and won't turn you into a weight watcher obsessed with scales. If you don't have a cup measure, which is equal to about 300ml or half a pint in terms of volume, use a mug – not filled to the brim – to give you an idea of what sort of amounts you should be eating.

Vegetables The word vegetable comes from the Latin verb 'vegetare' to enliven or to animate – an emotion not normally associated with a potato or a carrot. But it is important to realise that vegetables provide the broadest range of nutrients in any food class: they are a source of vitamins, minerals, cancer-fighting phytochemicals, water, carbohydrates and some protein. It is worth experimenting with different vegetables to find ones you like. Try to have more green leafy ones, and fewer starchy vegetables such as courgettes, tomatoes and onions. Limit yourself to one to two servings of starchy vegetables such as beetroot, potatoes, parsnips, sweet potato and pumpkin.

Fresh is usually best, then frozen, then canned. Eating more vegetable portions a day can be quite daunting, so don't be discouraged. Vegetable soup is a good way to achieve your daily intake: made with an onion, spinach and/or leek, for example, it can easily amount to three vegetable portions. Have carrot sticks and some hummus as a morning or afternoon snack. Then have vegetables with your evening meal; one cup of leafy greens, and a salad could easily account for two to three portions. You'll find you won't be hungry, and rather than thinking about what you *can't* have, think of what you *can* have and you'll soon find you won't have room at the end of the day for that bar of chocolate. Aim for: five portions

One portion equals:
1 cup raw leafy vegetables
or
½ cup non-leafy cooked vegetables

Fruit Fruit is a source of simple sugar, fructose, which the liver has to convert to glucose, so try to stick to a limited amount. Go for a range of coloured fruits to take advantage of all the vitamins and phytonutrients available. Again fresh is best as cooking may destroy some vitamins. Fruit is a useful snack and dessert. Aim for: three to four portions a day

One portion equals:
1 medium fruit
or
½ cup of cut-up fruit
or
¼ cup of dried fruit

Also eat in season; seek out fruit and veggies from local food shops and farmers' markets. Fresh, locally produced fruit and vegetables, plucked out of the ground down the road, taste better than those flown from half way round the world – think how you feel after a long flight.

Caffeine and Alcohol Try to limit alcohol – women to no more than two units a day and men to three units – and spread alcohol consumption out over the week. The calories in alcohol have no nutritional value – i.e. no vitamins, minerals, fibre, fat or amino acids, just sugar. Processing alcohol puts a strain on the liver, interferes with sleep and damages brain cells. Caffeine plays havoc with blood sugar levels, making you crave sweet foods, interferes with sleep and stresses the adrenal glands. Both caffeine and alcohol can cause mood fluctuations and deplete vitamins, especially the B vitamins.

Have a Nice Healthy Day!
Breakfast: 100g oat-based muesli, soaked in orange juice with a portion of fresh fruit such as a slice of pineapple, chopped

cherries, grated apple, topped with natural yoghurt and pumpkin and sunflower seeds.

Benefit: lots of complex carbs with the muesli as well as fibre, plus fructose from the fruit, protein from the nuts, seeds and yoghurt, and some good fats in the seeds and nuts.

Snack: roasted soya beans – these taste like and are even nicer than peanuts to nibble on.

Benefit: great source of protein and fibre and carbohydrate all rolled into one.

Lunch: big bowl of spinach, coconut and lemon soup with an oatcake.

Square of chocolate.

Benefit: the soup is an easy way to get about two to three servings of vegetables, plus a source of iron and vitamin C. You could add nut butter or some cottage cheese to your oatcake for extra protein – there is some in the coconut. It's nice to end on something sweet at the end of a meal and dark chocolate will not have too high a GI to send your blood sugar rocketing, especially as it will be consumed with a meal.

Snack: carrot sticks and hummus.

Benefit: a good way to increase your vegetable consumption, as well as enjoy the benefits of chickpeas and tahini, both of which are good protein and carbohydrate sources.

Evening meal: chicken, coriander and peanut rice noodles. Apple and blackberry crumble.

Benefit: lots of protein, carbohydrate and flavours in this spicy dish. The almonds and oats in the crumble add some protein and complex carbohydrate to this fibre-rich fruit-based pud.

Drink: 1.5 litres of water throughout the day – herbal teas count.

Exercise: at least twenty minutes to get your heartbeat up

enough so as to feel it thumping – hoovering, hanging out the washing and getting off the bus a stop early count as well as time spent at the gym.

Bonuses: enough energy to get you through the day; you won't feel tired, you will be less likely to hit the biscuit tin, in a better mood, and better equipped to deal with stressful situations – better outlook, happier and you will sleep better.

Eat Well with Nell Is User-friendly

Dip in – you have permission to read the chapters that interest you the most or are most relevant – losing weight perhaps, or eating for a marathon, or good mood food. The last chapter is about foods that are worth getting fat for. I love food, but a little bit of saturated fat won't hurt most people, so don't live a life of denial. Enjoy a little ginger and mascarpone cheesecake then run/cycle it off or have a healthy day the next, and don't beat yourself up about it – just handle the recipes at the back with care, but the rest are suitable for everyday eating, so mix and match.

Feeds How Many?

I have tried to use manageable amounts of ingredients in recipes, i.e. whole tins or whole vegetables and whole fruits so you are not left with half a pepper or a whole bunch of celery minus one stalk sitting in the fridge. The recipes are geared for one person to four-ish, so if you have cooked food left over, freeze it and you will have your own supply of 'ready meals'.

Quantities and Measurements

For spices and herbs, these can only be a rough guide – they lose their pungency over time. They are also dependent on the ground they are grown in and even the strength of the sun. When we were filming *The Woman Who Ate Scotland*, we featured The Really Garlicky Company, based near Nairn in the north-east of Scotland. I learned that Scottish garlic has a lovely soft flavour as it ripens gradually under the long, but not intense Scottish sun, whereas garlic from nearer the equator will be sharper as it has been blasted by a more unforgiving sun. New garlic in the spring is gorgeously soft, juicy and strong but as the year progresses it gets drier and less powerful. I don't want to make cooking even more complicated – factoring in how much sun your clove of garlic has or its age – but experiment with quantities. Add more garlic if you like it; if you don't, leave it out. Most dishes can cope with a bit of variation. If you have an extra pepper or an onion, add it. Equally if you love basil add some more. Hate coriander seeds? Leave them out – or add another spice. Measurements only really matter when you are baking. You need to taste as you go along, so see whether you need to add any extra spices or balance another flavour.

A knob of butter definitely doesn't mean a doorknob; it means enough butter to melt or lubricate whatever you are cooking. A 'knob' should weigh about 25g, so weigh it once, then you have an idea what a 'knob' looks like.

Fresh ginger – again it is hard to measure amounts – gets less pungent as it gets older. I like ginger, so I tend to say use half a thumb's-worth, that is from the tip of my nail to the nail bed, but you might find that much too hot, so use less and build up. Ginger is a great antiseptic and anti-inflammatory, and can quell nausea and motion sicknesses.

Tasting

Digestion starts before you even get your forkful of food near your mouth. Just the thought of food and your salivary glands literally 'water', getting ready to digest incoming food. Thinking about food, then preparing, chopping, tasting, stirring are all actions which are part of the cooking process. I wrote a piece for the *Hong Kong Standard* asking whether there was a correlation between the quality of a chef's food and his/her girth. I discovered that most chefs I interviewed had a tendency to put on weight, as they said they tasted as they cooked. One chef admitted that he never tasted the food; he was the only thin one.

The Buddhists believe that you should think positive thoughts while cooking and think about the people for whom you are cooking. Such was my interest in Indian food that I volunteered to work in the Hare Krishna kitchen in Hong Kong to get authentic recipes. There I learned to make puris and veggie curries and lentil stews, but no food could be tasted until it had been blessed, and no swearing or bad thoughts were tolerated in the kitchen. I saw the chef drop a whole plate of chopped tomatoes on the floor and he just smiled beatifically. The Hare Krishna food was fantastic and I think it is why I will always prefer home-cooked food over restaurant food. If a friend/relative has cooked food for you it is a major effort and should be appreciated. A chef in a restaurant does care, but doesn't know you and, as much as he or she appreciates your custom, has to think of the bottom line and portion sizes. I cannot say how strongly I feel that it is important for you to get into the kitchen and cook – use simple seasonal ingredients if possible, as well as convenience foods, but above all revel in cooking for you and your friends. And unless you have strong Buddhist principles, taste as you cook. And add salt and pepper at the end of cooking, as sometimes salt can make food tough.

Convenience Foods

By convenience foods, I mean foods that are convenient to buy and use for cooking. The ultimate convenience foods in an ideal world would be those you can find in the garden; pick some green, sprightly non-bolted rocket or reach for your spade and dig up some perfectly formed carrots and, with a shake of organic soil, they are ready to eat.

Sadly this is a dream for most people who lack a garden, time or inclination. I had a small share in an allotment and it was sheer joy to cycle to my vegetable patch, pick my rocket against the backdrop of Edinburgh castle and pedal back home with bundles of the peppery stuff. Sadly in real life, when it's pouring with rain and guests are coming round in half an hour, it's more convenient to go to the corner shop and buy a bag of 'ready-washed'. Next best thing to growing your own is the pleasure of going to a farmers' market or local produce shop, then you know you are buying locally and in season. Hopefully the person selling was involved in the growing or buying process and can dispense helpful cooking hints.

Although supermarkets usually have an extraordinary display of fresh fruit and vegetables from round the world, sometimes they fail; you'd set your heart on making spinach and ricotta cannelloni, but they are out of fresh spinach – maybe it'll come in tomorrow? Or you're going to try making mango salsa to go with grilled chicken and there is no way the hard green oval shapes in front of you will ripen by the evening, so being able to buy or stock up on frozen spinach or frozen mango can really de-stress your shopping and cooking life. There is a place for foods that are frozen or tinned in your kitchen, that is foods that are convenient to buy, store and use. In most cases, the peeling, washing and chopping has been done for you.

But I do think you should buy fresh when you can as there is a therapeutic pleasure – and often a sensuous one – in preparing food yourself. Rinse a pile of fresh crisp spinach leaves, steam and watch them distil like magic into a small dark green mass of tangled leaves, giving off a sweet, slightly bitter smell which invites you to taste, and then season them with a pinch of freshly grated nutmeg. There is no way you can compare this to opening a tin of spinach only to be confronted with a soulless, acrid pile which no amount of lemon juice or nutmeg can restore to its former green glory. The joy of gnawing the flesh off the mango stone after having cut the flesh into chunks is also one that freezing denies. However, there is definitely a place for convenience food in today's cooking and eating, and courtesy of the freezer door and store cupboard it means that there are so many more recipes – and indeed nutritious dishes – at your fingertips.

Power to the Freezer

Freezing can often be a most efficient way of getting produce straight from the field to your plate. I know a farmer in Fife whose broccoli is picked on a certain day; the lorry arrives and takes his and other farmers' broccoli straight off to be frozen within three hours of picking, which is very impressive. Professional freezing is fast, the water in the food is converted into tiny ice crystals, so that bacteria have no chance of gaining a foothold and spoiling the food. Rapid freezing also lessens the chance of damage to texture or flavours. Freezing has little impact on nutrients and often frozen food is higher in vitamins than fresh which has had to endure hours of transportation and storage. Vitamin C, which is water soluble, is very susceptible to damage and often frozen food will have a higher content than fresh. Use frozen food as soon as it has defrosted as vitamin C will continue to decline.

Although freezing is very handy for vegetables and out-of-season fruits, I have to draw the line at frozen apples. Apples are easily available and life cannot be too short to peel – no, not even peel, but simply to cut an apple into slices. It is no slower than taking that forlorn box of peeled and sliced Bramleys out of the freezer and leaving to thaw in a pool of sad apple juice.

> Few things are quite as soul destroying as thawing gravy when you were expecting chocolate sauce

Freezing is also good for leftovers or batch cooking, and means you can always have a homemade pasta sauce or your own 'ready meal' on hand. But home freezing also means you have to be organised. Buy freezer bags and a proper freezer pen. You will revel in thinking 'I am a domestic god/goddess' as you label your home-cooked food and pop it in the freezer, but don't make the mistake of thinking 'I'll remember what it is'. You won't and few things are quite as soul destroying as thawing gravy when you were expecting chocolate sauce.

Tins

Tins are packed with the prepared food and topped up with syrup, oil or brine. The food is heated, the lids are sealed then sterilised to kill bacteria. Some vitamins are lost, especially vitamin C, but ironically enough, the canning process preserves and in fact improves the uptake of others such as beta-carotene (which makes vitamin A in the body) in tinned carrots and lycopene (an antioxidant which can protect against prostate cancer) in tinned tomatoes and the lutein (good for skin and wrinkles and eye health) in tinned spinach. Tinned fish such as sardines and anchovies are good as canning softens the bones which are a good source of calcium. Be wary of tinned tuna, however, as any omega 3 oils will have been destroyed and regular consumption of tuna can cause mercury build up. Tinned pulses are so much more convenient than soaking and boiling dried pulses. Tinned fruit tends to be soaked in syrup, so be selective. On the whole tinned vegetables and pulses and small boned fish are useful allies in the kitchen.

Vitamins and Minerals

Food should be your main source of vitamins and minerals, not supplements; too many supplements or an imbalance can cause problems. Vitamins and minerals come naturally balanced in your food. Vitamins are organic substances that activate enzymes to speed up all biological reactions such as the maintenance of healthy bones and the control of hormone activity and energy release, and you get them through food. Minerals are inorganic – they come from rocks and ore – and get into the food chain via the soil. So by eating plants that have grown on mineral rich soil, or animals which have grazed on the soil, you can get the minerals your body needs for its chemical processes. Nowadays food has become so over processed and soil levels are so depleted, that it is harder to get optimum levels. Supplements can have therapeutic effects, but they are powerful, so I would recommend taking professional advice from a nutritionist.

Shopping List

I've put together a list of foods and flavourings that are always handy to have in your kitchen, so you can rustle up a meal or have the base for a meal.

Tins: tomatoes, chickpeas, beans, coconut milk, sardines, anchovies

Fill your freezer: soya beans, green beans, broad beans, spinach, corn, peas, all kinds of berries and frozen fruit

Jars: tahini (for making hummus and mixing with yoghurt to make a vegetable topping); nut butters: peanut, hazelnut, almond and brazil

Sea salt and whole black peppercorns

Sugar-free muesli – buy or make your own

Seeds: pumpkin, sesame, sunflower seeds, linseeds for soaking and adding to cereals

Nuts: brazil nuts, almonds, peanuts, pecans, hazelnuts, cashews

Dried fruit: dark brown non-sulphur dried apricots, figs, raisins, dates

Grains: brown rice, millet, pearl/pot barley, quinoa, oats and pinhead oatmeal

Pastas: wholemeal, quinoa, spelt and other non-wheat pastas

Pulses: red and green lentils, split peas

Breads: rye, spelt, quinoa, barley, sourdough; keep them sliced in the freezer, so you can quickly defrost and have with a nut butter and banana for a fast blood-sugar sustaining snack

Flours: spelt flour, wholemeal flour, oatflour, soya flour

Spice: cinnamon, cumin (ground and seeds), ground ginger,

chilli powder, turmeric, coriander (ground and seeds), curry powder, whole nutmeg

Stock cubes – veggie bouillon is better, try and avoid monosodium glutamate and salt cubes with added salt

Oils: sunflower oil and standard olive oil for cooking, extra virgin for salads; flaxseed, hemp, pumpkin and sesame seed oil for adding omega 3s to spreads, dips and salads

Eggs – good for making fast meals like omelettes and scrambled eggs; try to buy organic and free range as they should have better flavour and more nutrients

Handy Kitchen Items

- Food processor. This is my favourite. They are not hugely expensive and are so good for grating, slicing and chopping vegetables that could take ages by hand and involve injury. Vegetables are important to healthy eating as they are a very rich source of fibre, antioxidants and vitamins and minerals. You are more likely to enjoy them if some of the hard work chopping them up has been done for you.
- Hand-held blender. Less washing up is required as you can stick the blender – which looks like a big wand – straight into cooked vegetables to turn to soup. Also great for whizzing up hummus in an instant.
- Pestle and mortar. Spices really jazz up dishes but need to be bashed about a bit to release their aroma and flavours. In some cases, spices have therapeutic qualities; cinnamon, for example, can steady blood sugar.
- Measures, scales, spoons and jugs – all can be bought cheaply and just make life easier.
- Muffin tins (non stick) are great for portion control; don't just

make muffins, but use them to speed up the baking process of bakes and cakes.

- Bamboo or metal steamer. Steaming is a great way to cook without losing the valuable nutrients to the cooking water. I have just borrowed an electric steamer for food demos, and it is a great new toy – it steams food so quickly and easily and collects the juice from the steamed food in a tray which you could use as stock. It has several compartments so you could steam a whole meal.

Losing weight

1

Be Careful What You Wish For . . .

Funnily enough, losing weight can be a case of 'be careful what you wish for'. In seven months I lost almost 10kg cycling 5,000 miles from Hong Kong to Sydney through lack of calories versus extreme exercise and a bout of food poisoning. I did not have model/stick-like legs; I still had tree-trunk thighs from all the cycling, however my bones stuck out on my neck, I seemed to have more wrinkles and there was no fun in trying on clothes – well, in West Timor you can only buy sarongs and you can't really ask if they come in a smaller size. I did not feel any happier, if anything I felt tired as I was under nourished and lacking in energy, so there is no point being a 'size-four' sarong – probably the equivalent of a tea towel – if you are too tired and unmotivated to go out for a drink, to go shopping or any of the things you dreamed of with your new imagined shape.

A more realistic wish is to be happy with your body shape,

to be brimming with energy and enthusiasm for life, to sleep well, have a strong immune system and not be dogged by colds and illness and to feel for most of the time in a positive frame of mind. This is what the road to good nutritional health and happiness can promise – and along the way you'll lose the pounds without really trying too hard or suffering.

Clients often come to see me because they want to lose weight. They feel unhappy with their appearance and usually there is another problem alongside the weight gain – constipation, stress or depression. Excess weight is also associated with so many other conditions and risks: heart disease, diabetes, gout, gallstones, sleeping problems and arthritis, so by dealing with excess weight, you also deal with so many other health-related issues – so you might never need to get beyond this chapter!

First the bad news: for long-lasting weight loss, it can't be fast. Speed diets or faddy diets don't work in the long run; I've tried them: cabbage, Atkins high protein, food combining etc.

The good news for long-term weight loss: forget the calories, throw away the diet foods, the reduced sugar and the no-fat foods. It is time to rediscover good no-nonsense food, which doesn't come with a list of ingredients your grandmother wouldn't recognise. Rediscover the joy of cooking and eating. It won't be quick, you should be aiming to lose about a quarter to half a kilo a week (a couple of pounds) but in a month that is two kilos (about eight pounds).

Too Rich, Too Blonde and Too Thin

So you want to lose weight, but how much? The most current measure is the Body Mass Index (BMI) which measures your height in ratio to your weight. To find yours, you can use one of the many online calculators; simply Google 'body mass index' and click on a site and type in your height and weight. A simple calculator-way is to divide your weight in kilograms by your height in metres and divide the answer by your height again to get your own BMI.

73kg ÷ 1.82m = 40.11 ÷ 1.82 = 22 which is a healthy BMI of 22.

These are the weight ranges, set by the World Health Organisation:

- If your BMI is less than 18.4 you are underweight for your height.
- If your BMI is between 18.5 and 24.9 you're an ideal weight for your height.
- If your BMI is between 25 and 29.9 you're over the ideal weight for your height.
- If your BMI is between 30 and 39.9 you're obese.

As you can see, these are quite wide parameters, and are very general. If you are very physically active or a professional sports person then your BMI could be beyond the recommended range. Muscle weighs so much more than fat, which means you might register as obese even though you were a perfect physical specimen. If you are using one of the online charts you can tap in another weight and see the wide spectrum considered to be a healthy weight. But it comes down to what you feel comfortable with. When I lost weight on my cycling trip, I would still have been in the healthy section, but I did not look that good – I looked scrawny and it hit me that I had always thought you could 'never be too rich, too blonde and too thin'. Now I was too thin and I suspect you can probably be too blonde and being too rich will have its own problems too . . .

Blood Sugar

The key to weight loss is managing your blood sugar or blood glucose balance. Take a look at the Tools Section on managing your blood sugar. It's eleven o'clock in the morning and you're feeling hungry, so you buy a chocolate chip muffin, and just as quickly as you grabbed it from the shelf and munched it without really thinking, in fact the moment it passes your lips, an enzyme called amylase in your saliva starts breaking down the carbohydrate into sugar – and there is a lot of simple sugar in a processed white flour chocolate chip muffin. The sugar solution, along with the rest of the munched-up muffin, descends into the stomach and intestines for further breaking down into protein and fat, vitamins and minerals – if there are any – and absorption.

But it's all systems go; your pancreas is kicked into action as it receives signals that incoming sugar is sending blood sugar up, so it produces the hormone insulin to help carry glucose from the blood into the cells via the liver. Then suddenly too much insulin is coursing through your veins, so what next? Your body receives signals that the blood needs more sugar to cope with the extra insulin. It needs sugar and fast, so you will have to drum up incredible willpower to say 'No, body, I've had my daily muffin' – now you are on a one-way ticket on the sugar roller-coaster. Any number of mental pictures of you in skimpy swimwear on a beach or photos of very fat people on the fridge door will make no difference; it is hard to override the strong signals from your body demanding more easy-to-access sugar to respond to the high insulin levels in your bloodstream.

> " You are on a one-way ticket on the sugar roller-coaster "

These fast-release sugars are high in calories, but don't fill you up, so it is incredibly easy to eat beyond your body's needs. The only way off this sugar roller-coaster is to manage the sugar cravings and switch to foods that will slow down the release of sugar and moderate your insulin levels into the bloodstream. So a major key to weight loss is maintaining a constant blood sugar balance throughout the day, and this will also prevent sugar cravings and bingeing.

It's Not Always Your Fault
Sometimes there is a problem and the body can malfunction. If you're a healthy weight and then experience sudden unexplained weight changes, you must go and see your doctor.

A mineral called chromium may help to manage sugar cravings. Chromium is required in trace amounts for sugar metabolism in humans as it makes the body more sensitive to insulin and can help get glucose into the cells. It is quite interesting that a diet of refined sugars, white flour products and lack of exercise actually depletes chromium levels – just when you need it most to help with high blood sugar caused by these products. Foods rich in chromium are rye bread, oysters, wheat germ, green peppers, chicken and apples.

Allies in the Fight for Weight Management

Complex Carbohydrates
Wholegrains: there are many wholegrains available so it's worth experimenting with them as you can use them as meal

accompaniments, salad bases, for thickening soups and they will also help balance sugar.

Barley: I love using barley either in soup or as an accompaniment. There are two kinds of barley available in the shops: try to get pot barley which is simply barley with only the outermost inedible husk removed which gives it a lovely nutty flavour. Pearl barley is more refined as it has lost both its husk and has been polished.

Brown rice: this has only had its hard inedible outer hull removed and retains its bran and germ. It takes longer to cook – about thirty minutes – than white milled and polished white rice, but for sheer filler value and taste I think it is worth it. Be careful about reheating rice as you may not kill off all the bacteria which can thrive at warm temperatures. You can freeze cooked brown rice and reheat, but I think it loses taste and texture.

Buckwheat: this is not a member of the wheat family but a grass and its seeds are ground to make a flour. The flour can be used to make fibre-rich pancakes and cakes; it too has a nutty flavour. Sometimes the roasted seeds are called kasha. The grains soak up flavour and you can add spices such as cumin and cinnamon to jazz it up. It is also a good source of protein.

Quinoa: pronounced keenwa or quin-noa, this is a South American grain which is very rich in protein, but low in fat and has some carbohydrate. Its small yellow grains have little flavour but an interesting texture. Cook quinoa in stock for about fifteen minutes, until the grains become opaque. It has a nutty texture and is very useful if you are making a veggie-based stew and need to add some protein to bump up the food values.

Bulghur wheat: this is fast – pour hot water over the wheat

grains and watch the grains swell. It is the main ingredient of the Middle Eastern tabbouleh salad along with parsley, tomatoes and lemon juice.

Oats: pinhead, medium and fine and jumbo oats all deserve a home in your kitchen. The big jumbo oats have been steamed and rolled whereas pinhead has still to be flattened and has so much more texture; make porridge with a mix of both to vary textures. Don't write off oats as a breakfast food; add them to fruit and veggie crumbles to get the GI index down – substitute half the flour for oats to make crumble topping.

Protein

Low-fat meat such as turkey and chicken and fish are good sources of protein. Dairy products such as milk and cheese are high in saturated fat, so use them sparingly. But live natural yoghurt is easier to digest and its good bacteria are essential for gut health. Eggs are also a good accessible source of protein. Soya too is a useful source of protein. Soya milk can be used instead of milk and tofu soaks up flavours like a sponge, so there is no need to cast it in the tasteless pile. I have just discovered soya beans (Birds Eye sell frozen soya beans) which actually make a great snack cold as well as when served as a vegetable. They can even be roasted and served as a pre-dinner snack like peanuts. When I was cycling across Myanmar, fresh soya beans were sold in little bags and I carried them as an emergency snack in my front pannier.

Nuts such as almonds, brazil nuts, cashews (in moderation) hazelnuts, pecans, pine nuts, pistachios and walnuts are great as snacks in their own right: a quick protein fix, rich in essential fatty acids, or added to dishes for taste and texture.

Seeds such as sesame, sunflower, pumpkin, flaxseed are again great on their own as snacks and also useful added to dishes for extra protein boosts and crunch, and they contain essential fatty acids.

Pulses – protein/carb combo

Beans: kidney beans, chickpeas, butter beans, aduki beans all come in tins, so are easy to use – they can be added to soups and salads or whizzed to make dips. The dried versions need to be soaked and boiled endlessly. I can't taste the difference and the texture value outweighs the effort.

Lentils: these come in all shapes and colours, red easily breaks down, whereas brown and green keep their shape – but swap them around in recipes.

Split peas: great in stews as they keep their shape, and in Indian dishes. They are also good sources of fibre.

Essential Fatty Acids

These are found in nuts, seeds and oily fish and all their oils. Essential fatty acids can reduce cholesterol, help reduce saturated fats, speed up metabolism and even make you feel full.

Fibre

Vegetables, pulses and wholegrains will fill you up, so less chance of feeling hungry, and will help slow down sugar release into your bloodstream. Fruit has some fibre, but can be high in sugar, so limit.

Exercise

Exercise increases the metabolic rate – the rate at which the body burns calories either resting or in action. The way to increase your metabolic rate is to build up muscle which needs more energy than fat cells. In fact muscles use fat as their preferred source of fuel. You need to do some exercise every day: twenty to thirty minutes to make your heart beat faster. Don't rush into it; build up gradually and as you lose weight you'll become fitter and able to do a bit more.

Quantities

Quantities are key to weight loss; a rough guide is the palm method as your hand size is relative to your weight and height. Cup your hands together as if they were a bowl you'd serve your food in, and this is the rough size of your carbohydrate serving at each meal.

The palm of your hand will give you a rough guide as to the size of your daily protein portion: two to three poached eggs depending on your palm. Imagine a pack of cards; that is the size you should aim for when deciding how much meat and fish to eat. And sorry, with cheese it should be a lot smaller – we're talking a small matchbox.

Try eating off a smaller plate, so it appears you have more. If you are having lunch or evening meal, not breakfast, your plate should be almost half vegetables. Don't rush back for seconds, wait twenty minutes and if you are still hungry, then you probably need more food, but your stomach takes time to tell your brain that it has had enough.

Other Diets

A big part of my job in Hong Kong involved eating, which meant going out to lunch and dinner regularly. Over the years I have tried different diets to try to keep my weight under control – and have to say the low GI diet is the most sustainable and makes the most sense.

> The low GI diet is the most sustainable

High-protein Diet

High-protein, low-carbohydrate diets such as Atkins work initially as your body is deprived of energy in the form of carbohydrate, so it has to break down protein to make energy – which is usually the body's last resort and not what it is best equipped to do. Excess protein stresses the kidneys and in the long term this diet will cause harm. Excess amounts of protein can make your body very acidic which is harmful to your tissues. Your body then turns to calcium to buffer this acidity, and it can only get this calcium from your bones and teeth, which puts you at risk of osteoporosis. When you return to your normal diet, your body composition has changed: there's more fat and less muscle now, so in the long run you could even put on the weight you have lost.

I tried the Atkins diet, ironically before I went trekking in Nepal. I was working as the magazine editor at the American Club in Hong Kong where I would tuck into an all-singing-all-dancing fatty Club breakfast of eggs and cream and bacon every morning, but still felt queasy and lacking in energy. Two weeks into the diet I went off trekking in Nepal – where pulses rule – and my poor body was put into a spin: loads of complex carbohydrates in the form of porridge, lentil-based dhal, veggie curries and very little animal protein. I did lose weight, naturally, through eating a complex carbohydrate diet, very little alcohol, lots of veggies and occasional treats such as apple pie, combined with exercise. The Nepalese diet is a perfect low GI regime and many people round the world naturally eat like this, in fact in the West we did too, before we started processing foods and taking short cuts.

Meal-combining Diet

This is based on eating proteins and carbohydrates at separate mealtimes. But foods are very rarely split into carbohydrates and protein; vegetables have protein, albeit very little, and pulses and some grains have a mix of both protein and carbohydrate, so trying to eat protein and carbohydrate separately is almost impossible. However, I like some aspects of the food, combining diet as it automatically makes you eat less. Take a typical meal of chicken with vegetables and potatoes – you don't need the carbohydrate potatoes, which are a source of fast-release sugar anyway, so just eat the chicken and veggies. Cutting back on the quantity of food will help weight loss, but the diet is not helpful in terms of overall blood sugar management.

Cabbage Diet

This one is hard work! You eat a base of cabbage and vegetable soup supplemented by protein and carbohydrates on different days. It works short-term, as you are eating fewer calories and are full of cabbage – i.e. fibre. But you will have no friends by the end and you'll begin to dread mealtimes. When you come off it you will have learned nothing new, and developed a long-term hate of cabbage, so it's not really worth it.

Diet foods
Reduced-fat Foods

I mistrust specially marketed low-fat foods. Often the manufacturers have added some kind of filler such as modified starch or even hydrogenated vegetable oil to add a pleasing creamy texture. Reduced-fat milk will have less saturated fat, so it is a good option, but be wary of having too much milk in your diet as excess dairy can trigger bloating, excess mucus, skin problems as well as weight gain.

Coconut milk contains good saturated fat that is easily metabolised to give your body quick energy and which also stimulates your thyroid. The principal fatty acid in coconut milk is lauric acid, which is also found in breast milk and is known to promote normal brain development and contribute to healthy bones. It is also less likely to cause weight gain than a polyunsaturated oil, so don't be tempted by the reduced-fat options.

Low-sugar Products

Again, what has the sugar been replaced with to make the food still taste appealing? Artificial sweeteners carry their own health risks, many of which are not proven, but they have been associated with cancer and changes to the genes. You may have seen fructose in the sugar section in shops and read the suggestion that because you need to use less of it, you take in less calories. Sadly this is too good to be true. It is true that fructose is a naturally occurring simple sugar, and amounts of fructose are found in most vegetables and fruits, but eating too much of this 'natural' sugar at once seems to overwhelm the body's capacity to process it. Instead of turning it into sugar the liver can't cope and long-term consumption of fructose can lead to elevated levels of both sugar and insulin.

Low GL Meals

To maintain a constant sugar/blood balance you need to eat

regularly, so aim for three to four meals a day – they can be small, but don't starve all morning, then hit the buffet table at lunchtime. Also it is better to eat well in the morning and gradually eat less throughout the day.

Breakfast

Breakfast is the most important meal of the day as your body is low in blood sugar when you wake up and needs fuel to get started. Many people say they don't have time for breakfast, but it really is worth it, if you want to stay strong and resist the temptations that lie ahead. So start the day with a mix of complex carbohydrates, good fats and protein, with some vitamins and minerals thrown in.

The most simple option is a smoothie (N.B. they're not perfect as more fibre would be preferable, but it is simple) – yoghurt (protein) whizzed with a banana (quick-release sugar carbohydrate packed with potassium) and a handful of oats (slow-release carbohydrate) and some crushed linseeds. You can even take this to work with you, so there is no excuse. Oat-based cereals are all good as oats are such a wonderful low-fat, slow-release source of energy. Muesli and porridge are all good variations. Avoid commercial breakfast cereals – just read the side of the packet and see how much sugar has been added. Many are wheat-based and wheat has become so over processed it has little goodness. Eggs with a carb such as rye toast and veggies such as spinach are also a good option, or a sweet potato omelette.

Snacks

Snacking is a good way to keep topping up blood sugar – try to create a protein, carbohydrate, good fat combo such as:

- Oatcakes with a nut butter or cottage cheese
- Apples, raisins and unsalted almonds or cashews
- Pumpkin and sunflower seeds
- Homemade oat flapjack made with seeds
- Homemade hummus and carrot sticks
- Homemade mackerel dip with crispbread
- Banana or cottage cheese on rye bread
- Dark chocolate and apple; the fibre in the apple and the protein in the chocolate help slow down the absorption of the sugar in both. This is a treat snack, so eat in moderation and resist eating the whole bar of chocolate at once!

Lunch

The midday meal should combine carbohydrate, protein, good fat and fibre. An ideal lunch would be high in veggie content: homemade soup is both filling and nutritious, especially if you add a tin of pulses for extra protein and fibre. Eat veggie soup with an oatcake and some nut butter for extra fibre, fat and carbohydrate. Soup is a good lunch option as it can easily be transported in a thermos or plastic soup bag and heated up. Sandwiches are an obvious lunch-on-the-move, but watch the wheat which can be fast GI and substitute it with a slower GI bread such as rye or quinoa bread. Finish with a piece of low GI fruit or low-fat yoghurt.

Evening Meal

Again the combination should comprise carbohydrate, protein, good fat and fibre. You don't want too rich a meal at the end of the day; grilled fish or chicken or turkey with salad or salsa perhaps to spice it up. Pulses such as lentil stew with veggies are good meals that can be made up in bulk, portioned and frozen then quickly defrosted. Stir-fry vegetable combos are good ways to get the veggie intake up, together with a whole-grain.

Recipes

Enjoy cooking; don't regard losing weight as a penance and don't be too hard on yourself. And don't try and change your eating habits overnight. Try a new breakfast one day, then a lunch, and build up, then you will have more chance of success. Eating breakfast is probably the one major key to weight loss, so really try and make sure you start the day with a carbohydrate and protein to help stabilise your blood sugar.

Porridge that's Worth Waking Up For

Oats are a superfood – they can help lower cholesterol, regulate blood sugar and are a great source of slow-release energy. Even if you think you hate porridge, it's worth trying it with these variations.

First, a basic recipe for making porridge. To enhance this complex carbohydrate breakfast, serve with natural live yoghurt or semi-skimmed milk, oat milk, etc. and top with sunflower or pumpkin seeds for added protein and good fats.

Serves 2

Ingredients

500ml water or 250ml water and 250ml semi-skimmed milk/ soya/oat milk

75g jumbo porridge oats and chuck in a few tablespoons of pinhead oats for extra texture

pinch of sea salt

Method

Bring the water to the boil, add the oats and simmer for 5–8 minutes depending on the thickness of the oats till cooked. Add the salt at the end so as not to toughen the oats.

Variations:

- Add a couple of chopped dried figs and a teaspoon of cinnamon to the oat and water mix
- Add a teaspoon of marmalade to the cooking porridge for a real breakfast feel
- Add a handful of frozen raspberries, blackberries or even mango to the cooking porridge
- To the cooked porridge, add a spoonful of apple purée made with two Bramley apples peeled and cooked with the juice of half a lemon and a dash of honey
- To the cooked porridge, add chopped fresh cherries and slivered almonds

Good-to-Go Banana and Nut Butter Toast

I love nut butters as they are an instant form of protein. The word 'butter' is used loosely here as nut butter is just unsalted nuts pulped to make a relatively smooth paste. Hazelnut, cashew and almond butters are a good source of protein as well as essential fatty acids. Rye bread – which has a higher GI and higher fibre content than brown bread – is quite hard going cut from the loaf, but toasted it takes on a delicious nutty flavour. The banana is high GI, but the nut butter and bread will slow the transit time down. This is a useful snack, when you feel yourself craving something sweet.

Ingredients

2 slices wholegrain/rye bread, toasted

2 tablespoons nut butter
1 banana, sliced

Method

Spread the toast with nut butter, pile sliced bananas on top and eat immediately.

Spinach and Eggs on Toast

Nutmeg-spiced spinach goes so well with creamy scrambled eggs and you need some toast to soak it all up. This is a great mix of carbohydrate, protein, omega 3 and vegetables; you can also substitute mushrooms for the spinach. Eggs are a good source of protein. What the hen eats goes pretty quickly into the egg, so of all the organic foods available, try to buy organic, omega 3-enriched eggs.

Ingredients

100g frozen or fresh spinach
whole nutmeg, grated to taste
2 slices rye bread
knob of butter

2 free range organic eggs
salt and pepper to season
1 tablespoon boiling water

Method

You can heat frozen spinach straight from the freezer, rinse fresh spinach and steam gently in its own water. Grate some fresh nutmeg onto the cooked spinach. Toast the rye bread. Add a tiny touch of butter to heat in a small saucepan. Beat the eggs in a bowl, season with salt and pepper and add a tablespoon of boiling water then pour into the pan of sizzling hot, but not brown, butter. Stir quickly with a wooden spoon till just beginning to set. Serve the spinach on toast and top it with the molten scrambled egg and season to taste.

Sweet Potato and Coconut Soup

Sweet potato is a great source of slow-release energy. If you peel the sweet potato you don't get the flecks of skin and you'll have a more sophisticated-looking soup, but the skin contains lots of fibre and there is vitamin C lurking just under it. Fresh ginger gives this soup a pleasant kick and the coconut adds a sumptuous richness.

Coconut milk is not the liquid found inside a coconut, but is made from grated coconut meat steeped in hot water – the flesh is then squeezed and the resulting white liquid is coconut milk. Coconut milk may also speed up your metabolism.

Serves 4–6

Ingredients

1 tablespoon sunflower oil
2 onions, chopped

500ml vegetable stock, made
with non-additive cubes such

2 cloves garlic, finely chopped
½ thumb fresh ginger, chopped
3 sweet potatoes (scrubbed if unpeeled), roughly chopped

as Kallo organic or Marigold Swiss Bouillon powder
400g can chickpeas, rinsed and drained
400ml can coconut milk

Method

Heat the oil and cook the onions till soft, then add the garlic and ginger and cook for a few minutes. Add the sweet potatoes and stir to coat with the onion mixture. Now pour in the stock, cover with a lid and simmer till the potatoes are soft. Stir in the chickpeas and coconut milk then blitz the soup in a liquidiser. Reheat if necessary.

Parsnip and Sweet Potato Crisps

If as a weight watcher you thought you were condemned to life without crisps, think again. These baked, spiced vegetable crisps taste far better than any you might buy, they're really easy to make – and they look good! Remember, veggie crisps will still have quite a high GI so don't binge on them, but if you're trying to lose weight they are far better for you and more satisfying than many varieties of mass-produced crisps. Experiment with other root vegetables, too – beetroot, carrot and, of course, potato. To slice the veggies into paper-thin discs, you will need a food processor with a slicing attachment or mandolin.

Serve with a fresh dip of yoghurt, chopped fresh mint and salt or, for a spicier version, try yoghurt with a dash of curry powder and a spoonful of mango chutney.

Serves 4 as a snack

Ingredients

2 sweet potatoes, scrubbed
2 parsnips, scrubbed
olive oil

1 teaspoon curry powder
sea salt (optional)

Method

Preheat the oven to 140°C/275°F/Gas 1.

Thinly slice the vegetables using a food processor/ mandolin. Put the sliced vegetables in a large bowl, add a glug of olive oil and the curry powder and toss to coat the slices. Rub olive oil over a baking tray and spread out the vegetable slices, taking care that they do not overlap. Bake in the oven for 40 minutes, or until crisp round the edges, turning once. Drain on kitchen paper and serve. If you wish, sprinkle over a little sea salt before serving.

For People Who Hate Vegetables: Roasted Garlicky Veggies

This is a great way to eat loads of vegetables; feel free to experiment with quantities and ingredients. Baked garlic is wonderful, it turns to a soft, mellow purée – so different from the raw clove. Should you have any left over, this dish freezes well.

Serve with nutty pearl barley or brown rice.

Serves 4 as a main dish

Ingredients

2 red onions, cut in thick

1 aubergine, sliced

wedges

500g courgettes or marrow,
cut in thick, diagonal slices

3 peppers – 1 red, 1 green,
1 yellow, deseeded and
roughly chopped

1 butternut squash (about 300g),
peeled, deseeded and cut in
wedges

250g fresh tomatoes, quartered

1 bulb garlic, divided into
whole unpeeled cloves

15g pack fresh thyme,
roughly chopped

75ml olive oil

1 tablespoon balsamic
vinegar

Method

Preheat the oven to 200°C/400°F/Gas 6.

Place all the vegetables and garlic in a large, deep roasting tin, sprinkle with the thyme, pour over the olive oil and stir gently to coat. Roast in the oven – stirring occasionally to ensure even cooking – for about 40 minutes, or till the vegetables begin to soften and turn golden brown.

If you like, you can hunt out the baked garlic cloves and, with the back of a fork, squeeze out their now soft, rich purée then mix it through the vegetables. Sprinkle on a dash of balsamic vinegar to finish.

Baked Aubergines with Tahini Yoghurt Dressing

This is a lovely, quick, protein-rich dressing and it goes so well with the earthy, smoky texture and taste of baked aubergines.

The dressing livens up lots of other vegetables, too. For example, it looks and tastes stunning over cold, sliced beetroot topped with fresh mint.

It's worth keeping a jar of tahini in the store cupboard. Tahini is made from sesame seeds, which contain protein, essential fats and vitamins, it also lends depth when added to *Hummus*, see page 94.

There are carbs and fibre in the aubergine so, if you want a light, balanced evening meal, this dish, along with a little green salad, could be ideal.

Serves 1–2 depending on size of aubergine

Ingredients

1 aubergine
2 cloves garlic, chopped
1 teaspoon sea salt
2 tablespoons tahini paste
500ml natural yoghurt

Method

Preheat the oven to 180°C/350°F/Gas 4.

Wash the aubergine and cut in half longways. Place on a baking sheet and bake till soft for about 30 minutes. Meantime, use a pestle and mortar to grind the garlic together with the salt. Transfer the ground garlic to a clean bowl and mix in the tahini paste and yoghurt to achieve a smooth, thick sauce.

Serve a generous dollop of sauce on top of the baked aubergines. The sauce will keep for a couple of days in the fridge.

Get-with-the-Beat Chicken with Mango Salsa

This mango salsa is a brilliant way to liven up chicken or fish and is so quick to make. Looks *do* matter on the plate and this colourful combination – vivid orange mango, green coriander and red chilli flecks – is very attractive paired with either a golden brown chicken breast or a white fish fillet.

Served with pearl barley – which contains protein, carbohydrate and fibre – this becomes a wonderful, low-cal, yet slow-release energy meal.

Serves 2

Ingredients

2 chicken breasts, skinned or
  2 white fish fillets such as cod or haddock

Mango Salsa

2 ripe mangos, chopped to bite-size chunks, or 500g mango pieces, defrosted
½ a red chilli, deseeded and chopped
juice of 1 lime

½ a shallot, finely sliced
handful of fresh coriander, chopped
salt and pepper to season

125g pot or pearl barley
600ml water

Method

First, make the salsa: toss the mango with the chilli, lime juice (reserve just enough to squeeze over the chicken/

fish), shallot and coriander and season with salt and pepper.

Next, cook the pot/pearl barley in 600ml of simmering water for about 30 minutes till it's soft but still has some bite. Most of the water will have been absorbed, but drain any residue. Prepare the chicken breasts/fish fillets. Wring out the last drops of lime juice from making the mango salsa over the chicken/fish and put the fillets on a lined grill pan under a hot grill, until cooked through and tinged golden brown on both sides.

Serve the chicken or fish on a bed of barley, topped with the gloriously orange and chilli red mango salsa.

Fresh or frozen mango?

In the freezer sections of larger supermarkets you can now find frozen mango cubes. They are superbly convenient compared to tracking down a ripe mango and the sticky and messy business of extracting the gorgeous orange flesh. Yet there is something incredibly sensuous about preparing and eating a mango, which bears no comparison to taking one out of a box in the freezer and leaving it to defrost for three hours. For ease, convenience and price, frozen mango wins, but occasionally buy a fresh mango and revel.

How to Prepare a Mango

I saw the barman at a pool bar in a hotel in Manila (where the bar is in the pool and you have an exhausting 10m swim over to the submerged bar stool) deftly prepare a mango thus:

Make a cut from top to bottom parallel to each side of the stone, leaving you with two outer sections and the middle section still attached to the stone. Run the edge of a tall robust glass against the inside skin of one half of the mango, so the flesh and the juice fall into the glass. Repeat with the other half. This way you get two perfect, smooth convex mango pieces. The middle bit which still has skin attached is the mango-cutter's treat, to be eaten with fingers. Let the juice run down your chin — now how can you compare that to defrosting frozen cubes of mango?

Spicy Lentils with Veggies

This is a lovely Indian dish made with red lentils and yellow split peas enlivened by a hot chilli and mustard seed sauce. I like the texture combination of yellow split peas – which don't break down – mixed in with red lentils which break down completely to make a rich base.

Serve with boiled brown rice to make this a complete protein meal. To bump up the vegetable input, you could dish up some fresh or cooked spinach on the side, or even chuck some spinach or cauliflower into the spicy lentil mix towards the end of cooking.

Serves 4

Ingredients

Spicy Lentils

115g red lentils
50g yellow split peas, called
   channa dhal, available in

½ thumb fresh ginger, chopped
1 tablespoon chopped fresh garlic
½ teaspoon turmeric
1 fresh green chilli, deseeded
   and chopped

Indian and healthfood stores   salt to taste
600ml water

Hot Sauce

2 tablespoons vegetable
  cooking oil
1 onion, sliced into rings
¼ teaspoon whole black
  mustard seeds

1 large dried red chilli,
  crumbled
6 cherry tomatoes, halved
fresh coriander, chopped,
  to garnish

Method

First, cook up the spicy lentils. Into a medium-sized saucepan put the lentils, split peas, water, ginger, garlic, turmeric and chilli, bring to the boil then simmer so that the mix gradually thickens, which takes about 10–15 minutes. Season with salt to taste.

To make the hot sauce, heat the oil in a frying pan and fry the onion with the mustard seeds and crumbled chilli for about 10 minutes till you have a mass of sweet, gooey onion rings. Add the cherry tomatoes and cook for a few minutes more. Spread the lentils onto a warmed dish, spoon over the hot sauce and serve garnished with chopped coriander.

Peppered Crusted Salmon

Topped with a hot, peppery caramel crust, this is a brilliant way to serve salmon – a good protein for weight watchers as the oily fish is rich in omega 3s which help balance hormones and stabilise metabolism.

Serve with a green salad, or with *Mango Salsa*, see page 59, or wilted spinach. It is quite a rich dish, so a light grain like bulghur wheat or couscous would go well, too. If it's just you, eat half and enjoy the other half cold the next day.

Serves 2

Ingredients

250g salmon fillet, skinned

Pepper Crust

1 tablespoon whole black peppercorns

1 teaspoon sea salt

2 tablespoons Muscovado or light brown soft sugar

2 tablespoons parsley, stalks removed

Method

To prepare the pepper crust, using a pestle and mortar grind all the ingredients till you have a rough, dark green mix. If you don't have a pestle and mortar, put the ingredients into a rounded bowl and grind with a rolling pin handle. Press the mix onto one side of the salmon.

Place the salmon, crust side up, on a foil-lined grill pan (it gets messy as the sugar caramelises and foil makes for an easy-to-clean pan). Cook under a hot grill then, when pink through the top half after about 3–5 minutes, gently turn over and cook the other side.

Puds

It is nice to end a meal on a sweet note but it can be hard finding puddings that are weight-loss and blood-sugar friendly – and which also hit the sweet spot. Fruit is good but can be high in quick-release sugars, so add a bit of fibre, and leave the skin on when possible. Add some protein to the fruit to slow down the sugar transit time, such as yoghurt or some sunflower or pumpkin seeds. Seasonal fruit salad with yoghurt and seeds sprinkled on top is a good end-of-meal option. You can always put a layer of yoghurt on top of a dish of fruit and sprinkle some demerara or muscovado sugar on top, then blast it under the grill until it is bubbling and serve it as a slow-release, waist-friendly pudding. If I have the will power I like to keep dark chocolate in the fridge and just have one or two squares to satisfy my sweet tooth. Chocolate at the end of a meal shouldn't send your blood sugar rocketing.

Roast Pears with Figs and Ginger

Out of season, it is always tricky finding ripe pears when you want them – and when you do, just eat them as they are. The beauty of this recipe is that you can use unripe, hard, woody pears because the gentle cooking renders them to a delicious softness. Figs, although high in sugar, are rich in fibre so they are a good slow-release energy fruit.

Serve the roasted fruits with yoghurt to add a touch of protein.

Serves 4

Ingredients

4 Comice pears, peeled,
cored and sliced

4–6 dried figs, chopped

½ thumb fresh ginger (or more
if you like ginger), sliced

50g demerara sugar

juice of 1 orange

Method

Preheat the oven to 180°C/350°F/Gas 4.

Combine all the ingredients in a mixing bowl, transfer to an ovenproof dish and roast for 25 minutes or till the pears are soft and golden.

Banana Ice Cream

This is a great recipe if you thought ice cream was off limits . . . Bananas are a high GI food but if you have this delicious, creamy ice at the end of a meal, or top it with yoghurt and some seeds, then it shouldn't send your blood sugar rocketing.

Serves 4

Ingredients

4 firm ripe bananas   Splash of milk

Method

Peel the bananas and wrap in clingfilm and freeze overnight. Allow to soften for 20 minutes before roughly chopping them up then blitz in a food processor till thick and creamy. You may need to add a splash of milk to create a smooth ice cream. Serve immediately or refreeze and allow to soften for 20 minutes before serving.

Lose Weight Checklist

- Eat regularly – don't skip breakfast and have something to eat every couple of hours.
- Make every meal and snack a low GI one – a little protein, good fat, carbohydrate and fibre.
- Watch your quantities – use your hand as a guide and don't go back for second helpings.
- Avoid all processed foods, biscuits, cakes, crisps – all sources of calories which will be high in sugar and hard to resist.
- Cut back on wheat-based products such as pasta and bread; eat more non-wheat complex carbs.
- Exercise – thirty minutes minimum to raise your heartbeat.
- Include essential fatty acids in your diet; even though they are a fat, they are a good saturated fat and can help speed up your metabolism, so include oily fish such as salmon or herring which also contain good proteins.
- Reduce alcohol as it is just empty calories.
- Water – drink a glass before a meal, to 'fill' you up. It might be a good idea, if you are eating out, to drink a glass of water while everyone is raiding the bread basket.

Have a Good Weigh-in Day!

Breakfast: have one 100g (or less) bowl of oat-based, muesli or porridge with fruit, yoghurt and seeds.

Benefit: oats will slowly release sugar into your blood-stream, and are a good calming base and you will enjoy protein and vitamins from the fruit and yoghurt.

Snack: eat ten parsnip and sweet potato crisps with yoghurt dip.

Benefit: parsnips are a good source of fibre which helps fill you up while the protein in the yoghurt slows down energy release.

Lunch: eat one bowl of sweet potato coconut soup and oatcake, or half an aubergine and yoghurt tahini with green salad.

Benefit: veggie soup is filling without piling on the cals, as is aubergine, while coconut and yoghurt are good protein choices, so you have a good base to get you through the afternoon.

Snack: have ten roasted soya beans.

Benefit: a little protein and carb make a good pick-me-up for the afternoon.

Evening meal: prepare 125g hot peppered salmon with half a cup of couscous and grilled courgettes, with a square of dark chocolate as a treat.

Benefit: salmon is a great protein but also a good source of omega 3s which help you lose weight. Fill up on veggies.

Exercise: take thirty minutes or more to speed up your metabolism.

Water: drink 1.5 litres a day or more if you have been exercising.

Bonuses: as well as losing weight you will feel and look better, you'll have more energy, be in a better mood, sleep better and be at less risk of heart and joint problems.

Exercise

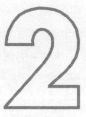

What to Eat to Get You Up that Final Hill

Hey ... slow down, don't skip this chapter – this is for anyone who does any kind of exercise, by which I mean any aerobic exercise; the kind that gets your heart pumping and brings a slight pink glow to your cheeks. Running for the bus does count, but if you follow the eating guidelines in this chapter, it might even inspire you to do more. Exercise has so many benefits, but these are the immediate ones: it can help with weight management and put you in a thoroughly good mood. Exercise also activates the immune system and it may prevent heart disease, osteoporosis and diabetes as well as lower blood pressure. I can't stress enough that if you want to feel well you need to do some kind of exercise every day. Equally if you want to run or cycle long distances then it is really important that you eat the right foods at the right time to maximise your performance and also enjoy the experience without damaging your body.

A good way to get regular exercise is to exercise with other people – join a gym and get the gym staff to devise a programme which involves aerobic and weight bearing exercises. Join in any of the group classes: Pilates, yoga, Body Pump etc. Join a walking or cycling group and go on regular organised walks and cycle rides – the benefits increase the more you go. With easy to access exercise, you meet new people and get to know your own area better.

Or sign up to take part in one of the many sponsored runs/walks/cycles organised around the country. You'll find it fun to train regularly for the event and, as there is a firm date, you will have a fixed goal to aim for, rather than just a whim 'to get fit'. Ask a friend to train with you.

Apart from aerobic exercise, where muscles rely on oxygen to convert stored glucose into energy, which in turn causes the heart to beat faster to get oxygen to the cells, men and women

> Exercise also activates the immune system and it may prevent heart disease, osteoporosis and diabetes as well as lower blood pressure

should do load-bearing exercises. These will enhance bone density, which is especially important after we reach our mid-thirties. Women don't have enough testosterone in their bodies to bulk up the way men do, so there is no risk of developing a glistening sculptured bikini body, unless you take some sort of testosterone-boosting supplement.

Start Small

Start with small distances and work up. My first proper run was a fun event at university. Six of us had to run 3km (2 miles) each. We ran in fancy dress as it was Easter and dressed as 'hot cross bunnies'. We had big cardboard 'hot cross buns' tied to our fronts and cotton wool tails attached to our bottoms and floppy ears on our heads. It did look quite good en masse, and we actually won the fancy dress prize and had our picture in the local paper – ironically getting more coverage than the actual winner. I found it quite an effort running the distance and I cannot put it down simply to having a huge bit of cardboard tied round my middle or keeping track of my cotton wool tail. I am definitely fitter now than I was in my early twenties, so age is no barrier to getting fit.

It wasn't until I went to live in Hong Kong that I attempted another run. This time it was 10km (6 miles) on the new airport runway. The old Tai Kak airport was a wonderful grip-the-edge-of-your-seat descent through skyscrapers – you could literally see what channel people were watching on their TV as you headed down to land in one of the most densely populated areas in the world. The new Hong Kong airport at Chep Lap Kok was built on reclaimed land. We ran 10km up and down the lovely smooth unused runways. There were quite a few people who could not resist pretending to be planes with arms outstretched – and I was one of them – running along the unblemished tarmac.

Sightseeing on the Run

I had started running regularly with a friend on a circular path which curved round the high hill called The Peak in Hong Kong. We soon found we could maintain a steady pace, while gossiping at the same time, then afterwards we would hit the local noodle shop – not realising that this was exactly what our bodies must instinctively have been craving – carbohydrates in a salty broth.

We soon decided we could attempt a half-marathon, 21km (13 miles), so signed up for the Beijing event. It started in Tiananmen Square and we knocked off a whole kilometre just running round the enormous square – then with 20km to go, we ran down the massive empty road off the square, which is normally teeming with cars, bikes and pedestrians, through the old city to the new bits, the high rises, that no tourist ever sees. After the run, we felt so pleased with ourselves we had a huge buffet lunch then went round the Forbidden City which was the imperial palace during the Ming and Qing dynasties (1368–1911) and the largest palace complex in the world. Just the walk – or the hobble – from the Gate of Divine Might to the Tiananmen Gate within the complex was almost one kilometre – nothing like being a glutton for punishment.

So why not turn running into a pleasure with an aim? Check out the organised runs in the world's great cities: they are a great way to see a place and parts you would never ordinarily see as a tourist.

Exercise Has to Be Fun

Then I heard about a wine-drinking marathon, where you drink wine as you run. I didn't think twice, and signed up straight away to take part in the Marathon du Medoc – 42km (26 miles) in Bordeaux, drinking wine from some of the most amazing châteaux and famous vineyards in France. It was like running through a very expensive wine list – Château Lafite-Rothschild, Château Latour, Château Lynch Bages etc. I had a friend who was a personal trainer and she devised a training schedule for me which involved running/walking every day, increasing the amount gradually until I could run about 30km (18 miles) a few days before I left for France.

Even though it is a proper marathon, people view it with a sense of fun; most of the 8,500 competitors wear fancy dress. A friend and I wore kilts and 'Jimmy' wigs – tartan hats with ginger hair which played 'Scotland the Brave' when you pressed the badge at the front. Spectators and competitors would shout '*levez, levez*' but they were not referring to lifting my legs higher to improve my running style, but to my kilt! In our kilts, we were in good company running with fairies, devils, doctors with patients on stretchers and famous painters who carried easels round the course. There were plenty of water stops as well as wine, pâté, cheese and bread stops. No fitness book would ever advise drinking alcohol while running – and I cannot say it will do anything to improve your running ability – but it is incredibly good fun; just drink extra water to compensate. One of my most surreal moments of the marathon was tucking into oysters with a glass of white Bordeaux chatting to a Dane dressed as a Flintstone, by the banks of the Gironde.

Remember, exercise really has to be fun, otherwise you won't stick to it and enjoy all the benefits.

Exercise – How It Works

When you start to make more demands on your body, your heart starts to beat faster to get more oxygen to the blood cells. The cells need oxygen to convert their stored glycogen into energy – this means more oxygen is being pumped to cells all over your body, including to your brain. To get the long-term benefits you only need to exercise about thirty minutes a day perhaps three times a week. All this blood pumping oxygen round your body means that all cells are bathed in oxygen – this boosts the immune system and stimulates hair, nails and skin cells to renew, so altogether you will look and feel fabulous. Exercising even moderately increases your muscle mass and these exercised muscles continue to burn more energy even when resting, so when you stop they still continue to demand more energy. By exercising you will have raised your metabolic rate – the rate your body burns up calories. Furthermore, exercise releases endorphins which are neurotransmitters produced in the brain which induce euphoria and reduce pain.

Fuel Supplies

Carbohydrates

Your body gets its fuel principally from carbohydrate which is broken down by the body into glucose which is stored in the body as glycogen. When blood sugar levels are low – during exercise or long gaps between meals, the pancreas produces another blood sugar hormone, glucagon, which stimulates the liver and muscle cells to release the stored glucose (glycogen) which will raise blood sugar levels. So it is important to work with your body to manage your body's sugar balance as you are putting extra demands on your body through exertion, and also using sugar to help the body to recover afterwards. Carbohydrate is the main fuel supply, but the body also gets energy from fat and protein in the diet, but these are less efficient suppliers, so we need to concentrate on carbohydrates in terms of fast-release (high GI) and slow-release (low GI) energy.

Protein

You need protein for repair and renewing tissues, and for making hormones and enzymes, so your body is constantly in a state of repair and renewal. Exercise can cause very slight to quite significant damage to the cells and muscle, so if you are exercising regularly, it is important that you eat foods that are high in lean protein such as meat, fish, pulses, grains, nuts and seeds.

Fats

There are good fats and bad fats. Bad fats tend to be the saturated animal fats which can cause weight gain without contributing anything significantly to the body. Good fats are the omega 3 and 6s – essential fatty acids which help speed up the metabolism, making it easier for oxygen to get to the blood cells and they are also anti-inflammatory. These fats are found in oily fish, nuts and seeds.

Fibre

Fibre found in fruit, vegetables, grains and pulses is useful as it slows down the speed with which glucose is released into the bloodstream, but athletes have to be careful and not introduce fibre too quickly into their diets as it can cause bloating and discomfort. To reap the benefits, start small with the lentils, until your body is used to digesting them.

Water

Water plays a huge part in exercise, as your body is about seventy per cent water. Blood is mostly water and your muscles, lungs and brain all contain significant amounts of water. Even slight dehydration can produce a serious downturn in performance through an increase in body temperature. Your body needs adequate fluid stores to produce sweat which evaporates and cools the body, and to keep vital organs functioning properly. Blood transports oxygen

> There are good fats and bad fats

to your cells, removes waste, and protects your joints and organs, so it is incredibly important not to become dehydrated. You lose water through sweating, but it is important not to wait to drink when you are thirsty; you should make sure your body is always well hydrated. So drink before exercise, during and after.

As a very rough guide, expect to consume about 500ml water per hour – more in very hot weather or if you are a big person. It's worth repeating what I said earlier: to check whether you might be dehydrated or not, look at the colour of your urine. Pale yellow is the usual colour, if it is darker yellow, then you should be drinking more water.

To see how much water you lose, weigh yourself before exercising at the gym and after and you might be surprised to see how much you lose. One kilo of weight equals about one litre of lost water due to dehydration and sweat. The general rule of thumb is to drink more water than you have lost, so if you have lost one kilo in weight, you will need to drink about one and a half litres of water to replenish the lost fluid. But of course you don't just lose water, you also lose body salts as sweat is salty which leads us onto all those sports drinks.

Sweat also causes potassium to be lost. Potassium works with sodium to maintain the balance of body fluids. Raisins, bananas, oranges and dried apricots are high in potassium – so they make good post-workout snacks, and are also good sources of sugar.

Sports Drinks

There is a whole sports drink industry with special names for their products – the key ones are isotonic and hypertonic. These will not only provide fluid quickly, but will also supply some carbohydrate. Experiment while training to find a brand you like or you can make your own: fill a water bottle with the ingredients below, and take it with you during exercise.

Isotonic

Isotonic drinks have a similar composition to your body's own fluids – carbohydrates and electrolytes – so they are absorbed at roughly the same speed. These drinks are good as they provide a balance between refuelling and rehydration. They are meant to be drunk before and during sport to top up water and salt levels. Here are the approximate proportions to make your own:

200ml of non-citrus juice such as cranberry, pear, pineapple or elderflower
1 litre of water
pinch of salt

Mix all the ingredients together and keep chilled.

Hypertonic

These water-based drinks are designed to replace lost salts and sugars immediately after exercise. The quickest way to do this is with a solution of sucrose. They are more concentrated than the body's own fluids so you should not drink them while exercising as they could cause dehydration, but they come into their own straight after exercise. Again, you can buy hypertonic drinks, but why not make your own? I love elderflower and if it tastes good, then you have more chance of drinking it.

500ml of non-citrus juice such as cranberry, pear, pineapple or elderflower
500ml water
Pinch of salt

Mix all the ingredients together and keep chilled.

Fizzy drinks and cola, or any drink containing caffeine should be avoided, as they may cause dehydration.

Getting Started

The same eating rules apply to eating and exercise, whether you are running your first 5km, regularly play a team sport, or are training for a long-distance cycle or marathon.

Before Exercise

The key here is to build up glycogen supplies in the muscles. Before you start exercising, eat a low GI meal at least three hours before you exercise, then a smaller snack before you exercise, so you have some slow-release energy constantly available.

Good pre-exercise snacks (up to thirty minutes before you start exercising, or in the gaps between playing if you are involved in a tournament where there are heats) include:

- One tablespoon of nut butter
- A handful of nuts, dried apricots and raisins

- One banana
- Fresh fruit with low-fat yoghurt
- One small flapjack – see recipe on page 98
- One small muffin – see recipe on page 97
- Marmite sandwich on wholegrain bread
- Cold pasta salad

Many 'special' exercise bars may contain just as much fat and sugar as your favourite sweet. It is better to stick to lower fat options like the above.

Carbo Loading

You may have heard of 'carbo loading' which is an eating regime which aims to build up glycogen stores to full capacity before exercise. This involves various combinations of excess exercise and adjusting carbohydrate intake to force your body to store as much glycogen as possible. It can, however, be hard to manage and the downside is that you may end up with not enough energy on the day. Best to carry on doing what you have been doing for your training and not give your body any surprises. Filling up on pasta is still a good night-before eating tactic and there will often be an organised pasta party the night before a big race or walk.

During Exercise

Exercising muscles need energy fast – the main source is glucose stored as glycogen in your body's cells. Your body can store enough glycogen to last you about ninety minutes of exercise. If you are doing more than ninety minutes, once the stored glycogen is burned up, your body can covert fat and protein to energy. This is not so efficient, so you need to take isotonic drinks or eat fast-release, easy-to-digest sugars such as bananas as you run/cycle/walk. So it is a good idea to drink water or an isotonic drink every ten to twenty minutes while exercising.

For longer distances taking more than an hour, I carry carbohydrate gels, a mix of fructose, water, amino acids, salts and vitamins and flavourings such as vanilla, strawberry, pineapple etc. You can buy them in sports shops and come in easy-to-carry one serving sachets. You can easily tear open the sachet and glug the gel while running or cycling. You must take the gel with about 200ml water per 40g sachet. The carbohydrate gels give you such a tremendous boost – in a sort of Asterix and his magic potion sort of way – you can almost feel the energy being zapped through your body.

After Exercise

You have about fifteen glorious minutes to eat high GI foods such as energy bars made with dried fruit and take hypertonic drinks high in sucrose. These increase plasma glucose and insulin concentrations which will make it easier for your muscles to get more glycogen back into the cells. After this small window it is back to low GI meals.

Suggested meals if you are training for sports events (recipes for most of these suggestions at end of chapter)

Breakfast
Oat-based muesli with yoghurt and banana
Porridge made with water or milk with seeds and yoghurt
Breakfast cereal with skimmed milk, fruit, rye toast and nut
   butter and juice
Homemade muffins with fruit, yoghurt
Fruit smoothies or fruit-flavoured yoghurts

Lunch
Homemade vegetable soup and roll or oatcakes
Pasta with chicken and vegetables
Baked sweet potato with cottage cheese
Wholemeal rolls with protein filling – chicken, hummus etc.

Evening meal
Steak and sweet potato gratin
Ricotta lemon pasta with peas and soya beans
Rice noodles with coriander and peanuts
Apple and blackberry crumble

Water – drink regularly throughout the day – the average recommended amount is one and a half litres. Also don't drink lots of water with your meal as it will dilute your stomach acid which will affect digestion.

Strategy for a 5km, 10km Walk/Run (less than ninety minutes)
The event shouldn't take you much more than an hour, so you will have enough glycogen in your cells, just drink water or your isotonic drink regularly through the run.

The Night Before
Pasta with a light protein – eat early so you don't go to bed digesting.
Drink plenty of water.

Whatever the distance, the same glycogen-storing principles apply, so before the run, eat low GI meals to build up glycogen in cells using the recipes listed here. Decide what you are going to eat on the day of the run and start eating it while you are training; don't eat something new on the day. Start practising your dietary and hydrating regime during training to reduce the risk of stomach upsets during the race.

On the Morning of the Event

You will need to take a light meal, then allow three to four hours for its digestion. You may find it difficult to eat because of nerves; in this case try a liquid meal such as a fruit smoothie, or a fruit yoghurt drink. Ideally any pre-event meal should be mainly carbohydrate and low in fibre, so that it does not cause a stomach upset. It is important to practise the pre-event breakfast during training to find out what works best for you.

After the Run

Drink your homemade hypertonic drink and eat a banana or flapjack immediately after the run. Then celebrate with a complex carbohydrate, protein, fat and fibre meal a couple of hours later.

Strategy for Long-distance Exercise – Marathon, Long-distance Cycle (more than ninety minutes)

Follow the above, except that when you start your exercise, replace fluids early on; don't wait until you become thirsty. Drink small amounts frequently so as not to upset your stomach. Start replacing fluids within the first thirty minutes of exercise, and aim to drink 100–300ml of fluid every fifteen to twenty minutes during exercise. An isotonic sports drink is an ideal way to refuel and rehydrate.

Ideas for fast-release carbohydrates during the event:

- 800ml isotonic sports drink
- Carbohydrate gel plus water
- Homemade flapjack
- Two pieces of fruit – cut up apple or orange in a Ziplock bag
- One banana
- Two handfuls dried fruit

Recipes

These are all geared to providing energy when your body needs it – slow release and fast release – immediately after sport. Include these recipes as part of your training, so your body gets used to digesting them. On the day of a race you will be nervous enough, so your body doesn't need the strain of having to deal with new foods and food combinations.

It's not bananas – listen to your body

Don't get too caught up in the science of exercise – a lot of the time your body will tell you what it needs. When I was doing my big pedal through Asia, I remember there were days when I craved banana pancakes or banana fritters or a banana smoothie. Bananas are a good source of quick-release energy, and they are also high in potassium which helps blood glucose be transported through the cell wall and improves carbohydrate metabolism by helping the muscles act efficiently. They are also rich in vitamin B6, which helps metabolise more proteins and helps make more red blood cells which transport oxygen to muscles. So perhaps my body was telling me it needed a bit of help.

Banana Porridge with Maple Syrup

The cooked banana is rapidly digested and will therefore give you immediate energy, whereas the oats will provide a back up with their slow-release energy to keep you going later on.

I find I don't need to add milk as the banana gives a sweetness. In place of milk I have a spoonful of maple syrup – its flavour goes brilliantly and it also gives an immediate bolt of energy.

Serves 2

Ingredients

500ml water
75g jumbo porridge oats
    and chuck in a few tablespoons
    of pinhead for extra texture

1 banana, sliced
pinch of sea salt
2–4 tablespoons maple
    syrup

Method

Bring the water to the boil, add the oats and sliced banana and simmer for 5–8 minutes till cooked. Add the salt at the end so as not to toughen the oats. Serve with maple syrup spooned on top.

Banana Pancakes

Banana pancakes are a traveller's staple in south-east Asia and no self-respecting backpackers' café would fail to have them on the menu. These pancakes remind me now of happy, sun-drenched moments anticipating, then tucking in to this delicious, hot, nutritious breakfast fuel. When I was doing my long-distance cycle in south-east Asia, sometimes I even ate them in the evening as they provide a calming carbohydrate at the end of an arduous day. These pancakes are so good when you arrive home after a long run, for example, and want to eat something hot yet quick to prepare.

The batter mix keeps in the fridge for a day.

Serves 2

Ingredients

100g flour
1 tablespoon sugar
125ml milk
1 egg

1 tablespoon butter, melted in the frying pan you're going to cook the pancakes in
1 teaspoon vanilla extract
½ teaspoon salt
1 banana, sliced

Method

In a mixing bowl, beat the flour, sugar, milk, egg, melted butter, vanilla extract and salt to a smooth batter the consistency of thin cream. Heat a large, lightly greased frying pan and, when hot, pour in the batter and tip the pan so that the batter entirely covers the bottom. Lay the slices of banana on top and cook over a medium heat until the pancake's edges crinkle. Flip over and cook for 1 minute more to colour the bananas and serve immediately.

Banana Smoothie

Smoothies are a great way to take in nutrients if you are feeling nervous – prior to your big event – and don't feel like eating or cooking. Bananas are a good base as they act as a thickener as well as providing all that fast-release energy.

Serves 1

Ingredients

1 banana
250ml semi-skimmed milk
  or soya milk

1 teaspoon honey
1 handful of porridge oats
1 teaspoon cinnamon

Method

Whizz up all the ingredients in a liquidiser. Drink immediately because bananas don't keep well.

Try these other smoothies-to-go . . .

250ml fresh orange juice, 1 banana and half a fresh pineapple
250ml fresh orange juice, 1 banana and 200g frozen mango

Get some iron in

Iron is important for people who exercise regularly as it is iron in the form of haemoglobin which helps the uptake of oxygen by the red blood cells. Iron is readily absorbed from meat, especially red meat, poultry, fish and liver and other organ meats. Iron is less well absorbed from non-meat sources such as cereals, oatmeal, rice, pasta, beans, peas, lentils, nuts, dried fruits, dark green leafy vegetables and egg yolks. Vegetarians, therefore, have to careful as iron from non-meat sources is harder to absorb. Both vegetarians and meat eaters can increase how much their bodies absorb iron by eating iron-rich foods along with vitamin C. Think watercress salad with fresh orange or spinach and lemon and coconut soup. Exercise does not cause lack of iron (anaemia), but anaemia makes it hard to exercise. Iron-rich foods have other benefits so if you suspect you are anaemic – pale face, pale nails, lacking in energy and always tired – make food your first line of defence; iron supplements alone may cause side effects.

Spinach, Coconut and Lemon Soup

This is a wonderful iron-boosting, vitamin C-rich soup and the creamy coconut milk lifts it out of the worthy camp into sheer deliciousness. A great soup to warm you up after a hard, wet day's walking or cycling.

Serves 4

Ingredients

1 tablespoon vegetable oil
1 onion, chopped
200g spinach, frozen or fresh
500ml vegetable stock, made
   with non-additive cubes such
   as Kallo organic or Marigold
   Swiss Bouillon powder

juice of I lemon
400ml can coconut milk
sea salt and black pepper
   to season

Method

In a large saucepan heat the oil and gently soften the onion. Add the spinach and hot stock and simmer for about 10 minutes. Stir in the lemon juice and coconut milk, season to taste then serve.

Steak and Sweet Potato Bake with Green Salad

This looks glorious on the plate: sizzling steak, bright orange potatoes and a pile of glistening greens. Steak is rich in iron and sweet potato provides lots of slow-release energy. Baked sweet potato has a lower GI than regular baked potato, so try switching from regular to sweet potato – both varieties are cooked in the same way.

A food processor with the appropriate attachment makes quick work of thinly slicing the sweet potato, but you can slice by hand.

Serves 2

Ingredients

2 sirloin or popeseye steaks
olive oil to rub

sea salt and ground black
pepper

Sweet Potato Bake

2–3 sweet potatoes,
  scrubbed
2–3 tablespoons olive oil
1 red chilli, deseeded and
  finely sliced

2 cloves garlic, roughly
  chopped
1 knob fresh ginger, peeled
  and roughly chopped

Green Salad

100g rocket or watercress
a splash of hemp or flax seed oil

small handful of sunflower
  seeds

Method

Rub the steaks all over with olive oil, salt and pepper and set aside.

Preheat the oven to 180°C/350°F/Gas 4.

Thinly slice the sweet potato then, in a large bowl, toss together with 2–3 tablespoons of olive oil plus the chilli, garlic and ginger. Tip the potato mix into a shallow, ovenproof dish, cover with foil and bake till tender (about 1 hour).

When you are nearly ready to eat prepare the green salad. Toss the leaves with the seed oil and sunflower seeds.

Put the steaks on a foil-lined grill pan under a hot grill

and cook for a couple of minutes either side for rare, or according to how well done you like your steak. Serve the steaks with the baked sweet potato and salad.

Pasta

Pasta is the athlete's friend, as it is so quick to cook and so convenient, but be wary of including too much wheat in your diet. Wheat can be inflammatory and too much can trigger allergies in some people. If you have Shredded Wheat or Weetabix at breakfast, then a sandwich at lunchtime and pasta in the evening, it can all add up to an overly pasta-intensive diet, so try and limit yourself to no more than one wheat-based meal a day. As well as wheat pasta, experiment with other pastas; they are still a good source of energy. Try buckwheat, quinoa, spelt and barley and corn pasta. I've just discovered multi-cereal penne made with barley, oats, millet and emmer wheat which has a lovely texture and nutty flavour. Pasta dishes can be eaten cold the next day – so useful to take to an event in which there are heats and you need fuel supplies in between them. Also, if you rely on sandwiches, try making them with non-wheat breads such as rye, spelt or quinoa.

Ricotta Lemon Pasta with Peas and Soya Beans

This is a fantastically quick-to-make pasta dish. And, if you keep pasta in your store cupboard and peas and soya beans in the freezer, it involves only a short shopping list. Here, you could use all peas but I like to include some brilliant-green soya beans. Soya beans are a good source of protein and soya is a phyto-estrogen which can help balance women's oestrogen levels.

You can freeze any unused sauce if you want to make this dish in smaller amounts.

Serves 4

Ingredients

400g multicereal penne pasta
500g mix of frozen peas
　and soya beans
juice of 1 lemon
3 tablespoons olive oil,
　or flax or hemp oil

500g ricotta cheese
black pepper, freshly ground
bunch of fresh mint leaves,
　roughly chopped
Parmesan cheese, freshly
　grated

Method

Cook the pasta according to pack instructions. While the pasta is cooking, put the peas and soya beans into a pan of boiling water for a couple of minutes, till cooked, and drain.

To make the sauce, mix together the lemon juice, oil, ricotta, pepper and mint to form a smooth emulsion. Add the sauce to the warm, drained pasta, peas and beans and gently toss.

Serve with grated Parmesan sprinkled on top.

Rocket Pesto Pasta

The leafy greens are packed with loads of B vitamins, the raw garlic has antibacterial and healing properties with inflammatory feel-good omega oils plus the cheese and seeds provide protein. All this combines with slow-release energy from the pasta. And, when the pesto hits the hot pasta on the plate, it smells so good, and it tastes so good, too.

The pesto will keep in a screw-top jar in the fridge for up to a week, but will last overnight without refrigeration, if you are somewhere where there is no fridge.

Serves 2

Ingredients

200g non-wheat pasta

Rocket Pesto

50g rocket

50g Parmesan cheese, freshly grated

50g pine nuts

4 cloves garlic, roughly chopped

60ml olive oil or omega 3 oil

sea salt

Method

First make the pesto. In a liquidiser or small food processor, whizz together all the pesto ingredients to make a gorgeous, thick, bright green sauce. Next, boil the pasta according to pack instructions till *al dente* (retains a bite to it). Drain the pasta, spoon onto warmed plates and top it off with a good dollop of pesto.

Chicken, Coriander and Peanut Rice Noodles

Rice noodles are brilliant if you are in a hurry: boil a kettle of water, pour it over these transparently thin noodles and you have a good source of medium-release energy within 5 minutes. The lovely mix of textures and flavours in this chicken, coriander and peanut combination goes extremely well with the noodles.

Fish sauce is very popular in Asia. It is made from fermented fish, but don't let that put you off! Used sparingly in place of salt here, the fish sauce adds a special dimension to this dish. I also love the mix of fresh herbs, lime and chilli in this lovely, light yet filling meal.

Make it vegetarian by simply leaving out the chicken and the fish sauce.

Serves 4

Ingredients

4 skinless chicken breasts
juice of 1 lime
2 tablespoons vegetable oil
250g rice noodles
250g roasted salted peanuts
1 large red chilli, deseeded
  and chopped
1 knob fresh ginger, peeled
  and grated

6 green spring onions or
  ½ onion, chopped finely
1½ tablespoons fish sauce
15g fresh mint, leaves chopped
15g fresh coriander, leaves
  chopped

Method

Lay the chicken breasts on a plate and sprinkle a couple of teaspoons of lime juice over them. Fry the chicken gently in a pan with a little of the vegetable oil till cooked through.

Meantime, put the noodles in a heatproof dish, pour on boiling water to just cover them and allow to sit for about 5 minutes.

In another frying pan, heat the remaining oil till hot and add the peanuts, chilli, ginger and onions. Cook for a couple of minutes then on a medium heat add the fish sauce, remaining lime juice and the herbs and cook for another couple of minutes.

Cut the cooked chicken into bite-sized pieces. Drain the cooked noodles, put them into a large serving bowl and then toss everything together and serve.

Indonesian Dynamo Fuel

Flores is just one of the very many islands, along with Bali and Lombok, which make up the archipelago that is Indonesia. The islands are volcanic and therefore extremely hilly – it was hard work crossing them on my bicycle. I ate this traditional stew in a mountain village on Flores and it was fantastic. It is also a very delicious source of slow-release energy. If you add a cup of vegetable stock to the cooking corn, coconut and potato stew, you will get a lovely thick soup.

Serves 1–2

Ingredients

265g can sweetcorn, drained   1 large sweet potato,

400ml can coconut milk   scrubbed and chopped

Method

Put all three ingredients in a pan and simmer with the lid on for about 20 minutes to create this warm, comforting stew.

Omega 3 oils

Oily fish and their oils, and nuts and seeds, are good for people who exercise as they make the cells more receptive to oxygen. These oils are also anti-inflammatory which is good if you have been over-exercising. Instead of olive oil in recipes, you can substitute flax or hemp seed oil. But don't cook with them as they are unstable. Read more about their amazing benefits in Chapter Five on hair, nails and skin.

Hummus

Chickpeas are a good source of slow-release carbohydrate and protein. Tahini is a paste made from sesame seeds. I like it as it adds a bit of depth and 'stickability' to the hummus but you can leave it out.

Use the hummus as a dip for toasted pitta bread sticks or for raw vegetables – cauliflower florets, cucumber and carrot sticks etc. – or use it as a sandwich spread.

Makes enough dip as a starter for 4

Ingredients

300g can chickpeas, drained
juice of 1 lemon
2 cloves garlic, peeled and
  roughly chopped
1 tablespoon tahini

1 teaspoon ground cumin
60ml hemp, flax or olive oil
sea salt to taste
fresh coriander, chopped,
  to garnish

Method

Put all the ingredients in a food processor and blend to a smooth paste (or put in a high-sided bowl and blitz). Transfer to a small bowl and garnish with chopped coriander before serving. If you are a fan of coriander, blend some into the paste – this also adds pretty green flecks to the creamy yellow dip.

Apple and Blackberry Nut Crumble

This is a good energy-giving pudding with vitamin C-rich fruit under a blanket of protein-packed, energy-giving topping. You can vary the fruits according to the season or to use whichever fruits you might have in your freezer.

Serves 4

Ingredients

Fruit Base

2 large cooking apples, peeled,   50g sugar
  cored and sliced   grated zest and juice
1 handful of blackberries (or other   of 1 lemon
  soft fruit), fresh or frozen

Nut Crumble Topping

125g plain flour   ½ teaspoon ground cinnamon
125g cold, unsalted butter   150g chopped brazil nuts
25g rolled oats   125g soft brown sugar

Method

Preheat the oven to 170°C/325°F/Gas 3.

In a shallow, ovenproof dish spread out the apples and blackberries. Sprinkle the sugar, lemon zest and juice over the fruit.

To make the nutty topping, put all the ingredients into a food processor and whizz till the mixture resembles large breadcrumbs. You can mix the topping by hand but if you do, stir in the nuts and sugar at the end of mixing so you don't get sticky fingers. Spread the topping over the prepared fruit and bake in the oven for about 30 minutes till lightly browned and crisp on top.

Apple and Raisin Cinnamon Muffins

Studded with potassium-rich raisins, these are easy to eat any time you need a quick fuel injection. They look great, too, with the cooked apple projecting iceberg-like, from each gooey-yet-light, spiced muffin.

Makes 12 muffins

Ingredients

100g self-raising flour
100g soft brown sugar
1 teaspoon baking powder
1 teaspoon cinnamon
from a whole nutmeg,
  a good grating

300g (about 2) cooking
  apples, peeled, cored
  and roughly chopped
50g raisins
1 egg
60ml vegetable oil

Method

Preheat the oven to 160°C/320°F/Gas 1.

In a large bowl, mix together the flour, sugar, baking powder and spices then throw in the chopped apple and raisins and toss to coat.

In a jug, beat together the egg and oil and pour into the dry mixture. Stir lightly to combine, but don't overstir – don't worry if the mixture looks a bit lumpy.

Fill 12 muffin cases in a muffin tray and bake in the oven for 20 minutes till risen, golden and slightly springy to the touch.

Apricot and Sunflower Seed Flapjacks

These are a source of fast- and slow-release energy: the brown sugar, golden syrup and dried fruit provide the fast release; oats and seeds the slow. Have a few bites before you start exercising and keep nibbling throughout. These flapjacks would also be good at the end of exercising.

Makes 10 small flapjacks

Ingredients

125g butter
100g brown sugar
1 tablespoon golden syrup
175g jumbo porridge oats

75g dried apricots, cut in small
  pieces using scissors
75g sunflower seeds
pinch of salt

Method

Preheat the oven to 160°C/320°F/Gas 1. Grease a square, 18cm tin.

Gently melt the butter, sugar and syrup in a pan. Remove from the heat and stir in the oats, apricots, sunflower seeds and salt. Spoon into the tin and press down with back of a spoon. Bake in the oven for 30 minutes till golden brown. Allow to cool, then cut into handy-to-eat squares.

Energy Checklist

- Eat low GI foods at least three hours before event.
- Eat an energy-rich low-fat snack up to thirty minutes before exercise.
- Drink water before exercise.
- During exercise keep fluids up and take fast-release energy snacks or gels if necessary.
- After the event, have fast-release snacks fifteen minutes straight after, plus hypertonic drinks and a slow sugar release meal, several hours later.

Have a Good Hill Walking Day!

I love going hill walking at weekends with friends – and I always volunteer to organise the food, then I know I'll get my favourites. It also ensures we'll have enough energy to make it off the hill and into the pub for some après walking. Here is a menu I created for a great horseshoe-shaped walk I did, staying at the Loch Ossian eco-youth hostel on Rannoch Moor where you have to carry all your provisions in and out with you – so light ingredients, easy cooking and limited washing up is key!

Evening meal: pasta and rocket pesto. This is easy to make at home, then easy to carry and needs minimal cooking – only one pan is required for the pasta. Pasta will be a good source of energy the next day as the body will store it as glycogen. Pesto is a good mix of green leafy greens, so lots of vitamin B there to help the uptake of energy, and the cheese and pine nuts are a good protein source to help rebuild cells. The omega 3 oil will help keep cells receptive to oxygen and calm any inflammation.

Treat option: red wine from a wine-box sachet. Bottles are heavy, whereas now you can buy perfectly acceptable wine in a box or one-litre sachets. The empty container is great for carrying water the next day – just rinse well. Red wine contains antioxidants and will help you relax – just don't have more than one glass!

Breakfast: fruit and nut muesli with bottled fresh orange juice, yoghurt and banana. Add any water to the juice left over in the bottle for extra liquid on the hill. Loads of complex carbs, protein and fast- and slow-release energy for the day ahead.

Lunch: homemade hummus and cucumber wholemeal rolls. Protein, fibre and grain meal with slow-release energy.

Snacks: fruit and nut chocolate for longer gratification, and homemade apricot and sunflower seed flapjacks for slow- and fast-release energy.

Water: three litres plus – in a day's walking the body uses up lots of water. If it's a hot day, you might need more.

Bonuses: speeded up metabolic rate, stimulated release of endorphins, thus better mood; less stressed, immune system boosted, so less likely to get colds. Glowing skin from all the oxygen flowing through body and good heart health; lower blood pressure and less chance of getting diabetes and developing osteoporosis.

Boosting Your Immune System

For Sneeze-free Winters, Happy Healthy Holidays and Long-term Good Health

It's hard to boost something you can't see. So far in *Eat Well with Nell*, you can lose weight and watch the needle on the scales go left, get fitter and see how many more kilometres you can cram into thirty minutes. As for your immune system, how do you know if you have boosted it? Is it worth boosting? Is it even worth reading this chapter? Yes, trust me, it is.

You know if your immune system is not at its best if you get more than two colds a year; if you get a cold, then you catch another one; if you get a scratch and it take ages to heal; if you feel tired and lethargic or you suffer from food allergies and always feel under the weather, or if your cold sores flare up constantly. If this is you, then your immune system could do with a boost. On a more serious note, chronic conditions and auto-immune diseases such as rheumatoid arthritis and cancer are more likely to gain a hold on somebody with reduced immunity.

Stress and poor diet are two major causes of a flagging immune system. You will discover lots of anti-stress lifestyle changes in the next chapter, but this chapter deals with food that supports the immune system, so you can enjoy better health, every day.

Building Immunity

Supporting your immune system is one of the most important steps in making yourself resistant to disease. A weakened immune system leads to infection, infection causes damage to your immune system which further weakens your resistance. By building up your immune system through healthy eating, you can help break that cycle.

The Immune System

The immune system is not one organ, like the heart or liver, it is a system of complex interactions involving different organs, structures and substances.

Your immune system is continually under fire and is round the clock fighting off disease, viruses, bacteria, fungi and battling cancer-mutating cells, and yet you are blissfully unaware of this gang warfare going on under your nose – or, in fact, literally *in* your nose. The cilia – the little hairs in your nose – are one of your first lines of defence, as is your skin which is rich in unsaturated fatty acids which kill bacteria; even your sweat has antibiotic properties. The tears in your eyes help wash away potential invaders; your saliva helps flush out microbes in the air or in food, and hydrochloric acid in your stomach kills off germs that have made it past the saliva. And even if these germs get beyond your stomach, good bacteria in your gut are waiting for them. All this is a function of your immune system and constitutes your body's first line of defence.

It takes a pretty determined bug, therefore, to penetrate this cohort of defence, and the next line of protection your body produces is found in the immune cells in your blood – your red and white blood cells. If something foreign to your body such as a chemical, bacteria, virus, or antigen – a dangerous pollen perhaps – gets through your body's first line of defence, then the white blood cells produce a specific antibody to neutralise the antigen and destroy it.

White Blood Cells

There are several types of white blood cell. Some engulf bacteria, and some are responsible for releasing histamine, which dilates blood vessels to allow more oxygen to the injured area and carry away toxins and waste products. Others are responsible for producing immunities – that is they develop antibodies in response to an antigen which has been detected in your body. Others are called killer cells and destroy cells which have become infected or could be cancerous.

As they play such a huge role in the immune system, white blood cells are used as one indicator of health; if you have just been fighting off an illness, then your white blood cell count will be lower. When someone has the Human Immuno-deficiency Virus (HIV) – the virus which attacks the body's immune system – the scale of the attack and progression of the condition can be measured by the white blood cell count. Normally, a person produces about 100 billion white blood cells a day.

Red Blood Cells

Red blood cells are also immune cells; their main role is to carry oxygen around the body, but they can also attract disease-causing organisms to which the white blood cells are then attracted. Like the white blood cells they are made in the bone marrow.

The Lymphatic System

This is a kind of cleansing system. It consists of an internal network of vessels which contain a clear liquid called lymph which carries defence cells round the body. There is no pump like the heart which moves blood round the body, so exercise and muscles are the main ways by which lymph is made to move round the body. Lymph nodes are located in the neck, armpits and groin and their role is to isolate infections and fight them – that is why they become swollen if you are ill and why a doctor will check your neck or armpits to see if your body is responding and fighting an infection.

The thymus, which is part of the lymphatic system, is a gland situated just above the breastbone. It shows immediate development straight after birth, and as you age it shrinks, as it is very susceptible to damage caused by stress, drugs, radiation, infection and chronic illness. When your thymus gland is damaged, its ability to control your immune system is compromised. White blood cells, which mature in the thymus, are the ones which develop immunity. The thymus also releases hormones which regulate many immune functions. The thymus also programmes new cells with your body's unique code, so your body does not start attacking itself.

Allergies and the Immune System

Sometimes the immune system gets it wrong – it mistakes a harmless food or pollen for an antigen and produces antibodies to zap it – this is known as an allergy. There are two kinds of allergy – a Type I allergy for example is a classic food allergy which provokes an immediate response such as swelling lips and itchy mouth, then rash and diarrhoea. A food intolerance or Type II allergy, for example, takes longer to develop and manifests itself as headaches, stomach aches, eczema, or aching muscles and joints.

Sometimes the body gets it badly wrong and attacks its own cells, this is known as an auto-immune response, and causes diseases such as rheumatoid arthritis where your thymus gland is no longer programming new cells with your body's unique code. People with an auto-immune disease may have to take immune suppressing drugs to try and stop the body attacking itself, which of course leaves them open to all sorts of other illnesses. So that is why, before you get to this stage, it is so important to look after your immune system.

What You Can Do to Support Your Immune System – EAT!

You are born with an immune system, and as you grow it develops. Each time you get an illness your body develops its own antibodies so that it can recognise them again. Thus immunity is constantly developing, which is why your body needs all the support it can get. Food plays a large part in providing nourishment for the immune system and cells are constantly being renewed and replaced; some of the white blood cells which kill antigens found in your body only live for about four days.

Your Number One Food Support: Antioxidants

Free radicals are formed by any kind of combustion or energy release such as cooking, radiating or burning food (that is why you should avoid the burnt sausage at the barbecue). Frying at high temperatures may damage the oil, producing free radicals. An antioxidant can prevent or slow down this process – that is why you put a squeeze of lemon juice (antioxidant) on cut fruit to prevent it oxidising. Antioxidants interact with and stabilise free radicals and may prevent some of the damage free radicals otherwise might cause.

Key antioxidant nutrients are vitamins A, C and E, zinc and selenium, and the primary source of these vitamins is found in food.

Vitamin A is important for the health of cell membranes; it helps maintain the integrity of the cell tract and lungs, and prevents nasties from getting into the body and viruses from penetrating the cell membrane. It comes in two natural forms: the animal form called retinol which is found in liver, egg yolks, milk and butter, and as a vegetable form known as beta carotene. You can find carotenes in highly coloured vegetables such as yellow and orange squash, carrots, sweet potatoes, red peppers, tomatoes and mangoes.

Vitamin C is the hero – the James Bond, the knight in shining armour of the immune system. Vitamin C is probably the single most important vitamin for the immune system as it is essential for the production of white blood cells which help develop the body's own antibodies. It is also involved in helping the immune cells to mature

> " Vitamin C is the hero – the James Bond, the knight in shining armour of the immune system "

and it can destroy toxins produced by bacteria. It can also calm down allergic reactions and subdue inflammation. Most people think 'citrus fruits' when they think of vitamin C sources, but vegetables such as broccoli, cabbage, kale, spinach, parsley, peppers and watercress as well as berries, kiwis, lemons, oranges and strawberries are all rich in vitamin C. It is water-soluble and your body cannot store vitamin C, so you need to keep topping up every day. It is easily destroyed; once you cut a cucumber you have lost half the vitamin C within three hours, so be wary of all those lovely-looking, ready prepared, chopped and grated salads you see in the shops.

Vitamin E helps the white blood cells function and is also good for building up your cell membranes, the body's first line of defence. It is a fat-soluble vitamin present in nuts, seeds, avocados, seed and fish oils. It works best if selenium is present.

Zinc is vital for normal thymus gland functioning – it helps make thymic hormones and protects your thymus from cellular damage. It is also needed to make protein for cell growth and to heal wounds. Oysters are incredibly high in zinc; good sources are also brazil nuts, wheat germ, pumpkin seeds and egg yolks.

Selenium helps the white blood cells make antibodies. Brazil nuts contain large quantities of selenium as do wholegrain bread, fish, shellfish, walnuts and dairy.

Lutein, another antioxidant best known for its association with healthy eyes, is abundant in green leafy vegetables such as spinach and kale.

Lycopene is a potent antioxidant found in apricots, blood oranges, tomatoes and papaya. Funnily enough, heating and tinning makes it easier for the body to access lycopene, so tinned tomatoes are a better source of lycopene than fresh.

Vitamin B6 enhances the white cells' ability to destroy disease-causing organisms; the thymus gland needs Vitamin B6 to function. B6 is found in wheat germ, bananas, chicken, fish, wholemeal bread, brown rice and green vegetables.

Omega 3 oils increase the activity of the white blood cells that eat up bacteria, so try to include omega 3-rich oily fish such as herring and salmon in your diet or with an omega 3 oil which you can add to salads or hummus or smoothies.

Probiotics

The word probiotic comes from pro meaning 'for' and bio meaning 'life' which is a pretty general definition, but the World Health Organisation (WHO) has taken up the term and defines probiotics as 'live micro-organisms which, when administered in adequate amounts, confer a health benefit'.

Your gut is full of good and bad micro-organisms. Probiotics trigger your gut wall to make specific bug-fighting antibodies that move into your bloodstream to help optimise antibody production and suppress harmful bacteria in your gut. They also help to break down food, thus providing a source of energy essential for the cells that line the intestines.

Live yoghurt is a natural source of good bacteria. Probiotic yoghurt is made by adding specific bacteria strains such as Bifidobacterium lactis (this bacteria in large numbers can increase white blood cell count) to warm milk, which is then fermented at blood temperature. The bacteria feed on the natural milk sugars (lactose) and release lactic acid as a waste product. It is the lactic acid which gives yoghurt its characteristic tang. This increased acidity causes milk proteins to tangle into a solid mass. The increased acidity also prevents the rapid growth of potentially disease-causing bacteria. When you buy yoghurt look out for ones that say 'live' or 'probiotic' on the label; it should also should name the bacteria present such as Lactobacillus acidophilus or Bifidobacterium.

People who are moderately lactose-intolerant and can't drink milk, can enjoy yoghurt because the lactose in the milk has been converted to lactic acid by the bacterial culture. This means that the work has been done for them and their bodies do not have to break the lactose down.

The Baddies That Attack the Immune System

- Sugar is the single most damaging food for your immune system as it reduces the ability of white blood cells to engulf and destroy bacteria.
- Alcohol can have the same effect as sugar, as alcohol can inhibit the beneficial activity of the immune cells. Good news though: one glass of wine has certain antioxidant effects, but don't go for the second.
- Smoking, like alcohol, depresses white blood cell activity.
- Caffeine in tea and coffee inhibits the absorption of vital nutrients and suppresses the immune system. It can also increase the amount of minerals excreted.
- Iron plays an essential role in the production of white blood cells and is involved in the synthesis of antibodies.
- Overweight impairs the efficiency of your immune system.
- Antibiotics kill all bacteria in the gut – good and bad. If you are on a course of antibiotics, take an acidophilus

supplement to replace any good bacteria which have been zapped.

A Cold-beating Strategy

You've followed all the advice, but still a bacterium or a virus has got a hold and you detect a sniffle – act now and you can lessen the effects and help your immune system fight off the baddies. Flu-like symptoms of headache, runny nose and slight fever are good! A high body temperature stimulates the immune system to produce more white blood cells; heat increases antibody production and intensifies the effect, and it also speeds up chemical reactions. A fever is the body's way of killing off bacteria, so go with it and hopefully it won't last too long. The danger in taking over-the-counter medicines such as anti-inflammatory painkillers to reduce the fever or inflammation is that you slow down these natural processes; you feel better and perhaps push yourself back on your feet before your body is fully recovered, leaving you vulnerable to another attack.

Rest, go to bed. Let your immune system do its work.

While you are resting:

- Don't force yourself to eat, but if you are hungry, go for complex carbohydrates, vegetables and fruit, especially berries which are high in antioxidants.
- Bump up vitamin C. Eat more vitamin C-rich foods – see recipes.
- Try and include spicy hot foods in your convalescent diet – forget the bland invalid food. Hot foods such as chilli peppers, hot mustard, radishes, pepper, onions and garlic contain substances called mucolytics which are similar to

over-the-counter expectorant cough syrups. These liquefy the thick mucus that accumulates in the sinuses and breathing passages, so don't hold back on the chilli or the garlic!

- Dairy – cut back on cheese, yoghurt and milk because they increase mucus production which is a breeding ground for bacteria.
- Avoid fatty foods which thicken the lymph fluids.
- Avoid sugary refined processed foods which will only suppress your immune system.
- Drink more liquid, so you can maintain a moist respiratory tract to repel viral infection. Drinking lots improves the function of white blood cells, but avoid sugary drinks – the big enemy of your immune system. A good drink is a few slices of fresh ginger and a cinnamon stick with some lemon in a mug of hot water.
- If your doctor has prescribed antibiotics (antibiotics only work on bacteria, killing the weakest ones first, then the stronger later, which is why you should take the whole course) take an acidophilus tablet to replace the good bacteria in the gut which the antibiotics will have killed along with the bad ones. Antibiotics also deplete vitamin B levels, so make sure you are eating lots of green vegetables and wholegrains such as porridge, berries and a little natural yoghurt while recuperating.
- Once you feel a bit stronger, take some gentle exercise, to get lymph fluid moving round your body to expel toxins.

Bug-free Holiday Strategy

Luckily you can do more for your health than just taking out an insurance policy and hoping for the best. Here are some simple nutritional tips for happy healthy holidays.

The key to good holiday health is having a healthy immune system. You will then be well equipped to fight off any colds or other viruses you pick up on the plane and abroad. A strong immune system will also boost healing, so a tiny scratch from sea coral will heal quickly, lessening the chance of infection.

- Take probiotic tablets before you go in order to maintain your gut in the best possible health to fight off any unfamiliar bugs that you should encounter. Look for one with equal ratios of L acidophilus, B bifidum and L bulgaricus with a strength of about 1.2 billion. Live yoghurt also contains some of these good bacteria, so don't forego eating it wherever you are, but the tablets have such a large number of friendly bacteria, your strong stomach acids won't destroy them all.

- Make yourself less popular with the mosquitoes; mozzies dislike bitter-tasting blood, so eat foods like chicory, endive and radicchio.

- Don't put your immune system to the test – avoid foods that have been allowed to sit at room temperature, as this is the most dangerous temperature for bacteria to breed. Be wary of meat, especially poultry, unless you are confident of the quality of the kitchen. But don't miss out on fantastic local dishes; street food cooked on the spot is usually fine as you can see it being cooked in front of you.

Some of the best meals on my travels have been street food: golden sizzling banana fritters in Malaysia, spicy duck and pineapple red curry in Thailand and local stringy white cheese and avocado quesadillas cooked on a grill in Mexico. Be very wary of rice dishes; reheated rice is a major cause of food poisoning. Avoid salads as they may have been washed in non-clean water, and also drinks with ice unless you are eating in a place you can trust. It is also best to avoid fatty foods as they are harder to digest, as are big meat dishes while spicy dishes can irritate the gut.

Recipes

There are quite a few Middle Eastern recipes in this chapter. I first became fascinated with Middle Eastern cooking when I studied Arabic culture at university. The flavours are so fresh and varied and there are so many inspiring recipes using pulses, grains, beans, seeds and fruits and vegetables, and also yoghurt. I was a member of the Arabic society and every term the society arranged a dinner to promote the society and raise money. Members would cook and I remember boiling vats of chickpeas to make hummus and chopping mounds of parsley to make tabbouleh. The seminal book was Claudia Roden's *Middle Eastern Food*. She has gone on to produce more updated editions and all are very inspiring.

One section of the university course was Arabic food culture and one night I was revising for an end-of-term exam with my flatmate, who was poring over a biochemistry textbook.

> 'Hot as hell, dark as night, sweet as love
> Hot as hell, dark as night, sweet as love'

I recited over and over again. 'What on earth are you learning?' she asked, looking up from a tangle of letters and numbers.

'How coffee should be served.'

I could see from her face that she could not believe we would both graduate with a degree from the same university.

DIY Yoghurt

Yoghurt has wonderful health benefits. It is a good source of protein, calcium and vitamin B12 and is especially beneficial for the immune system due to its probiotic qualities.

A yoghurt-maker for the home is basically a container which you place in a slightly larger container with a heating element. In the long run, it works out cheaper than buying commercially produced yoghurt.

You don't need a special yoghurt-maker to make yoghurt. In her books on Middle Eastern cookery, Claudia Roden offers tips which include putting a bowl of fermenting milk in an airing cupboard wrapped in two shawls – but what happens if someone storms in searching for a clean towel . . . ?

You can use any kind of milk: evaporated, skimmed, goats, soya, full fat – each will add a different flavour to the end product. I prefer UHT milk, because if you use fresh, pasteurised milk you need to boil it first to kill off any bacteria.

Makes 1 litre of yoghurt

Ingredients

1 litre UHT milk
2 tablespoons dried skimmed
   milk powder (optional, but
   makes the yoghurt thicker)

1 generous tablespoon natural
   probiotic yoghurt

Method

Turn the yoghurt-maker on. Gently mix together the milk and dried milk powder in the yoghurt-maker then gently stir in the yoghurt. Put the lid on and leave for about 8 hours – the longer you leave it, the more sour it becomes as more of the lactose turns to lactic acid. When you take the lid off, it's like magic – the thin milk has turned to a rich, thick, white custard with a thin trickle of whey on the top.

Chill in the fridge to stop fermentation and eat within four days. You can now use the yoghurt you have made as the starter for your next batch.

If you want thicker yoghurt, strain your lovely new homemade yoghurt through a sieve lined with a thin tea towel over a bowl for about 1 hour. From 1 litre of milk, you will get about 500ml of thick yoghurt which you can use as you would Greek yoghurt. You can see how concentrated Greek style yoghurt is, and why it is more expensive!

More Things to Do with Yoghurt

In the West we have just cottoned on to the health benefits and cooking potential of yoghurt but in the Middle East and Far East, they have been enjoying yoghurt for centuries.

Labneh

I first tasted this garlicky 'cheese' dip in an Egyptian restaurant where it was served with warm pitta bread as part of the mezze. You can also serve it spread on oatcakes or as a dip with carrot and red pepper batons. The ultimate immune-boosting 'cheese' dip.

Makes enough dip for 4

Ingredients

2 garlic cloves, chopped

1 teaspoon sea salt

chopped herbs, such as parsley,
    mint, coriander, basil, to taste

2 tablespoons olive oil

500ml strained (thick,
    Greek-style) yoghurt,
    or see page 114

Method

Add all the ingredients to the strained yoghurt and stir
to combine.

Lassi

In the West, lassis have been re-branded as yoghurt smoothies.
A traditional Indian lassi is a yoghurt and either milk- or water-
based drink. In India, lassis are served either sweet or salty. On
a hot day a salt lassi, made from yoghurt, water and salt, is
incredibly thirst quenching – the original isotonic drink!

On a cautionary note, as in all things, moderation is the key.
I love banana lassi and, once, I consumed many before setting
off on a camel ride in the Indian desert. Eating too many
bananas can make you constipated and, bouncing around on a
camel's back for two days, I suffered just that. My doctor friend
was no comfort, telling me unsympathetically that it was my own
fault for being so greedy.

Serves 1

Ingredients

3 tablespoons plain,
    natural yoghurt

cardamom (snip the green
pod in half, scrape out and

flavouring of your choice: add the tiny black seeds)
    honey, salt, lemon juice,   150ml water or milk
    chopped banana or mango,

Method

Put the yoghurt and flavouring into a large jug. Gradually add the water or milk and whisk till smooth – a hand blender is very useful here.
    Serve cold in a long glass.

Garlic is a source of vitamin B, C and selenium but it really comes into its own for its immune-boosting properties, thanks to its sulphur-containing compound, allicin – this is what gives garlic its pungent odour. Allicin has been shown to be effective not only against common infections such as colds, but also flu and stomach viruses. Garlic is at its most powerful when raw, so add to a dish towards the end of cooking, rather than at the beginning.

Warts and All I once treated a stubborn wart on my finger with raw garlic strapped under a sticking plaster and within two days it had completely gone – whereas the commercial wart medicine had made no difference at all.

Really, and I Mean Really Garlicky Chicken (40 cloves)

When we were filming the TV series *The Woman Who Ate Scotland* we visited the Really Garlicky Company, a garlic farm near Nairn in the north-east of Scotland. The owners, Glen and Gilli Allingham showed me the young garlic shoots poking their heads up toward the Scottish sun.

The Allinghams explained that because the north of Scotland benefits from so many hours of daylight during summer, the garlic grown there matures gradually and this lends it a lovely, mellow flavour.

When we went to Gilli's kitchen to make this chicken dish I couldn't believe the amount of garlic she added, but it works, so don't hold back. Really Garlicky Chicken is such a satisfying dish to make – it smells gorgeous while it's cooking and when you take the lid off the casserole the rich aromas of garlic, herbs, wine and chicken are divine. And it's great fun squishing the cooked garlic under the prongs of a fork to release its fantastic flavour.

The Allinghams diversified from growing potatoes to growing some garlic and Glen said that since they started farming and eating garlic the family very rarely suffer from colds.

Serves 4

Ingredients

1 small (1–1.2kg) free range chicken

4 tablespoons extra virgin olive oil

40 (approx) garlic cloves, separated from the bulb but not peeled

juice and rind of 1 lemon

1 onion, chopped

handful of fresh herbs – flat leaf parsley, tarragon, chervil or basil, chopped

150ml dry white wine

salt and freshly ground black pepper

Method

Preheat the oven to 180°C/350°F/Gas 4.

Heat 1 tablespoon of olive oil in a large, lidded, heavy-based casserole dish and cook the chopped onion until just beginning to soften then add half the fresh herbs.

Lay the chicken on top of the herbed onions and scatter the garlic cloves around it.

Pare the rind from the lemon using a potato peeler and add to the chicken along with the squeezed lemon juice. Pour the white wine and the remaining olive oil around the chicken then scatter over with the remaining herbs and season with salt and pepper.

Put the lid on the casserole dish and place in the oven for 1 hour then remove the lid and cook, uncovered, for a further 20 minutes to brown the chicken.

Remove the chicken and carve. Pour the garlicky juices over the meat to serve – part of the fun of this dish is squishing the juicy cloves from their skins as you are eating. Creamy mashed potatoes are an ideal accompaniment as well as some steamed vegetables.

Inulin is a type of starch which passes through the stomach and duodenum undigested so it is able to stimulate the growth of bacteria in the gut by providing a good source of food for the resident bacteria. Inulin also promotes the growth of bifodobacteria — bifodobacteria is the primary organism found in mother's milk. Echinacea also contains inulin. Jerusalem artichokes are one of the richest sources of inulin.

Jerusalem Artichoke and Carrot Soup

No relation to globe artichokes, Jerusalem artichokes are available from October to March. The knobbly tubers should be smooth and clean; avoid any very lumpy ones and any that are limp and spongy. To prepare, don't peel, just scrub the tuber as there is lots of goodness close to the skin.

Before you rush off to boost your immune system with inulin-rich Jerusalem artichokes, the downside is that they can cause flatulence so mix these lovely tubers with another vegetable so you can enjoy the flavour and benefits. Here, artichokes and carrots combine to create a gorgeous, velvety soup and the carrots help to mediate the less attractive attributes.

Serves 4

Ingredients

1 tablespoon olive oil
1 onion, chopped
500g Jerusalem artichokes, scrubbed and roughly chopped
500g carrots, scrubbed and roughly chopped

1 litre vegetable stock, made with non-additive cubes such as Kallo organic or Marigold Swiss Bouillon powder
1 clove garlic, finely chopped
strained (thick, Greek-style) *DIY Yoghurt*, see page 114 and chopped parsley to garnish

Method

Heat the oil in a pan, add the onion and cook till soft then add the vegetables and cook for five minutes. Pour in the hot stock and simmer for about 20 minutes or till the vegetables are soft. A few minutes before the end of cooking time add the chopped garlic.

Blend in a food processor, reheat if necessary and serve with a dollop of yoghurt and a sprinkling of parsley.

Per gram, parsley contains more vitamin C than any other vegetable or fruit. Parsley is also rich in folic acid, and iron and also a good source of minerals and fibre. Both the Italian flat leaf and the curly vivid green have the same properties. Parsley also has a high chlorophyll content which means it can inhibit the negative effects of fried foods and garlicky breath!

Gremolata Does Lentils

There is nothing cheesecloth and sandals about this lentil recipe. Gremolata is a zingy mix of fresh parsley, lemon rind and garlic which can be used to jazz up a wealth of dishes including soups, grilled chicken, meat stews, fish and pulses. This handy taste enlivener is also a great way to access loads of immune-boosting vitamin C in lemon and parsley and immune-strengthening properties of raw garlic. Gremolata is best used fresh.

Serves 2

Ingredients

Gremolata

4 tablespoons fresh flat leaf or curly parsley, finely chopped

rind of 1 lemon, finely grated (use unwaxed lemon if possible, if waxed wash in hot water)

2 garlic cloves, finely chopped

Lentil Base

2 tablespoons olive oil
1 onion, chopped
1 carrot, sliced
1 sweet potato, scrubbed and chopped in chunks
75g green or brown lentils

425ml vegetable stock, made with non-additive cubes such as Kallo organic or Marigold Swiss Bouillon powder
175g standard mushrooms, sliced

Method

First make the gremolata by mixing all the ingredients together. Set aside.

For the lentil base, heat 1 tablespoon of oil and fry the vegetables on high heat for 3 minutes. Once the veg have browned, add the lentils and hot stock and simmer for about 20 minutes till the lentils are soft. In a separate pan, fry the mushrooms in the remaining oil till browned and soft then add to lentil mix.

Sprinkle the gremolata on top to serve.

Tabbouleh

Bulghur wheat (cracked wheat) is the classic base for this lovely, fresh-tasting, Middle Eastern salad. I, however, love the nutty flavour of pot or pearl barley and I like the idea of harnessing all those valuable B vitamins and selenium in the barley.

Bulghur wheat is ready to eat in 10 minutes, while pot and pearl barley can take up to 30 minutes.

Serves 4–6 as an accompaniment

Ingredients

300g pot or pearl barley
(or bulghur wheat)
600ml salted water
80g parsley, leaves only
20g mint, leaves only
juice of 2 lemons
100ml olive oil

3 spring onions, finely
chopped
6 tomatoes, skinned,
deseeded and chopped
in small chunks
sea salt and freshly ground
black pepper

Method

First, add the barley to the salted water and simmer for about 30 minutes then drain.

While the barley is cooking, finely chop the parsley and mint leaves (a small food processor is ideal for this) then put into a large serving bowl along with the lemon juice, olive oil, spring onions and tomatoes. Give the mix a light stir to combine then add the still warm drained barley and season with salt and pepper. Give another light stir to combine then let the tabbouleh sit for at least 20 minutes to soak up all those lovely fresh flavours before serving.

Oysters have the highest concentration of zinc of any food and are a good source of vitamin B12. As well as promoting healing, zinc is essential for the proper action of testosterone – a key nutrient in sperm production – so that could be one reason why they have such an aphrodisiacal reputation! But oysters aren't just for the men; women need zinc and testosterone too, though in smaller amounts.

The tricky bit is slicing the muscle that keeps the shell shut. Hold the oyster in your palm with the hinge towards you and with a flat bladed knife or oyster knife work the blade between the shell halves into the small opening near the hinge and twist until the hinge gives. Slide the knife along the top shell to sever the hinge muscle and remove the top shell along with any grit or broken shell. To get full nutritional benefit, don't cook them; I like them best just eaten as they are, with perhaps a dash of Tabasco or lemon juice.

Grilled Smoked Oysters with Spinach

Zinc and iron from the oysters plus vitamin C from the parsley and spinach which will help your body absorb the iron, make this one easy nutritious immune-boosting snack.

Serves 2

Ingredients

50g butter
½ small onion, finely chopped
1 clove garlic, finely chopped
1 tablespoon fresh parsley, chopped
50g frozen chopped spinach

50g fine wholemeal breadcrumbs
85g tin smoked oysters, drained
25g Parmesan cheese, freshly grated

Method

Preheat the grill to its hottest setting.

Melt the butter in a frying pan. Fry the onion, garlic and the parsley for 2–3 minutes until the onion has softened. Add the spinach and cook until it wilts. Add the breadcrumbs and cook for 1–2 minutes. Chop the smoked oysters in half and stir in. Grate the cheese over the mix and place under the hot grill to melt and brown the cheese. Serve immediately.

Immune-Boosting Store-Cupboard Pasta Sauce

This immune-boosting meal is quick and easy to make from ingredients which are basic store-cupboard essentials: tins or jars of oysters, clams and cockles (all are rich in selenium and zinc); tinned tomatoes (a better source of antioxidant lycopene than fresh tomatoes; garlic and onion (both rich in allicin and natural antibiotics).

Top off the sauce with masses of freshly chopped parsley and no virus should even think of coming near you.

Serves 2

Ingredients

200g wheat or non-wheat pasta
1 tablespoon olive oil
1 onion, chopped
400g can plum tomatoes
100g jar cooked cockles or
    clams, drained and rinsed

2 cloves garlic, chopped
at least 1 handful of parsley,
    chopped
50g Parmesan cheese,
    freshly grated

Method

Cook the pasta according to pack instructions.

While it's cooking, heat the oil in a large frying pan, add the chopped onion and cook for about 5 minutes till soft. Add the tomatoes and shellfish and simmer till you achieve a gooey stew, about 15 minutes. Add the chopped garlic and cook for a couple more minutes then add loads of chopped parsley and serve with grated Parmesan.

Chicken Liver Pâté

I have happy childhood memories of eating grilled liver with fried onions but if I ask clients to include liver in their diet they look unconvinced and say, 'I'll try'.

Chicken liver is a very economical protein as it is rich in selenium and vitamin A and is relatively cheap. Eating chicken liver as pâté is a tasty, non-threatening way to access all its goodness. Serve the pâté on thin slices of rye toast, oatcakes or warm brioche.

Serves 4 as a starter

Ingredients

50g butter
1 onion, finely chopped
2 cloves garlic, chopped
2–3 sprigs fresh thyme

400g chicken livers (use organic if possible)
600g mushrooms
lemon juice or brandy to taste

Method

Melt the butter in a large frying pan, add the onion, garlic and thyme, stew for about 10 minutes, then add the livers then gently cook for about another 10 minutes. Add the mushrooms and cook for another 5 minutes.

Remove the thyme sprigs and whizz in a food processor until you have a smooth, creamy pâté. Add lemon juice to taste – this cuts through the slightly metallic flavour of the liver – or, for a richer more robust flavour, add brandy to taste.

Creamy Coconut Brazil Nut Curry

Brazil nuts are an excellent source of selenium, so you will certainly get your day's supply with this easy recipe. You can vary the vegetables depending on what's available from your greengrocer or in your freezer.

Serve with brown rice or pot barley to soak up the lovely creamy, nutty sauce.

Serves 2–3

Ingredients

3 tablespoons vegetable oil

1 onion, sliced

1 clove garlic, chopped

2 teaspoons medium-hot curry powder

100g brazil nuts

400ml can coconut milk

2 courgettes, chopped in small chunks

1 small cauliflower, cut in small florets

125g broccoli, cut in small florets

Method

Heat the oil in a frying pan and gently fry the onion, garlic and curry powder for 5 minutes.

Put half the brazil nut kernels in a food processor and grind to a pulp. Add the ground brazil nuts and coconut milk to the pan and stir to make a creamy sauce.

Add the vegetables to the sauce and simmer until cooked but retaining some crunch. Roughly chop the remaining brazil nuts and stir through just before serving.

Fruit Salad full of Eastern Promise

Sugar is the enemy of the immune system, but sometimes it is nice to end a meal on a sweet note. Berries and brightly coloured fruits are very high in antioxidants so they are always a good bet on the pudding front.

To try and cut back on sugar, opt instead for flavourings which give a note of sweetness such as cinnamon, cardamom, ginger or rosewater.

I love rosewater, which is very common in Middle Eastern and Indian cooking. A few drops give a hauntingly sweet aroma. You should be able to find rosewater in the baking section of any large supermarket or deli.

Here, the fruit is served in a thin, sugar syrup, which is complemented by the sweetness of the rosewater. Vivid orange mango chunks contrast with glistening, jewel-like raspberries – a very pretty pudding.

Serve with strained (thick, Greek-style) *DIY Yoghurt*, see page 114.

Serves 3–4

Ingredients

50g sugar
100ml water
150g frozen raspberries

150g frozen mango
½ teaspoon rosewater
25g slivered almonds, toasted

Method

Very gently, heat the sugar and water till the sugar is completely dissolved. Add the frozen berries and mango to the syrup then add the rosewater. Remove from the heat and allow to cool. Serve topped with slivered, toasted almonds.

Immune-boosting Checklist

- Make sure you are eating lots of wholegrains, nuts, seeds and brightly coloured fruits and vegetables.
- Boost good bacteria in your gut with natural yoghurt or take a probiotic supplement.
- Vitamin C is the single most important vitamin for the immune system so try and make sure you have some fresh fruit at breakfast, homemade vegetable soup at lunchtime and perhaps a filling salad in the evening. Get in the habit of snacking on fresh fruit and carrot and red pepper sticks.
- Cut back on sugar, honey, fruit and refined foods.
- Exercising for twenty minutes, three times a week is a great way to keep lymph fluid moving and beat stress.

Have a Nice Immune-boosting Day!

Breakfast: muesli soaked in orange juice with yoghurt and fresh fruit – a vitamin C-rich start to the day with fruit and good for the gut bacteria from the yoghurt.

Snack: handful of brazil nuts and almonds – keep up selenium levels thanks to the brazil nuts eaten with vitamin E-rich almonds.

Lunch: tabbouleh – vitamin C rich-parsley with vitamin B-rich barley.

Snack: red pepper and carrot crudités with hummus protein-rich dip with vitamin C-rich veggie sticks.

Evening meal: garlicky chicken with roast sweet potatoes and green salad – loads of immune-boosting roasted garlic, protein-rich chicken to build up cells and there is some beta-carotene – good for cell membranes – in the sweet potato.

Fruit salad with yoghurt; antioxidant-rich fresh fruit and some probiotic yoghurt to end the day.

Bonuses: as well as not catching every bug going, enjoy lots of energy; your skin, hair and nails will benefit from the extra selenium, and vitamin A will neutralise those free radicals which might damage collagen, while vitamin C will build up more collagen plus your heart and blood vessels will benefit from the extra vitamin E.

Coping With Stress 4

While writing this chapter, I was giving nine food demonstrations at Taste of Edinburgh, a wonderful four-day food festival which takes place on the Meadows – a huge green space under the benevolent shadow of Edinburgh castle. The event is great fun, but also due to its nature quite last minute – I was cooking where, only a few days before, people were lolling on the grass. I had to bring all my ingredients and most of my utensils. As well as cooking demos, I was doing food and wine matching. Food I know lots about, but wine matching, slightly less. Despite having been to many wine tastings and collecting wine certificates, my knowledge has been blurred by far too much enjoyment of the fermented grape. Even though there was a lot of work preparing talks, sourcing food, organising equipment and begging friends to act as helpers, I didn't find it stressful; if anything I found it exhilarating and challenging.

Two days before the event, however, I went to a new hairdresser to have my hair cut and blonded – I am still subscribing to the theory that you can't be too blonde; thin and rich are still work in progress. I found the three hours in the hairdresser's chair incredibly stressful; my heart was beating faster, I had clammy hands and a dry mouth and felt anxious. I found it hard to believe that getting my hair done would be more stressful than giving food demonstrations to hundreds of people in a field. But stress affects people in different ways, so it is important to face your particular stress demons – not someone else's – and learn to confront them and make them irrelevant to your life.

Writing this chapter has helped me; just as I finished writing and researching it, and was about to send it off, my laptop died. Of course I hadn't saved the file. Was I stressed? No, I thought, I won't panic; I'll take it to a computer expert; I'll borrow a friend's laptop. The worst that will happen is that I will have to rewrite the stress chapter. It might even be better second time around and, do you know, I quite wanted a new computer anyway. As it happened, the computer man sorted the problem, all was well and I hadn't lost sleep, comfort-eaten or even felt more than a slight heart palpitation – but I am being more vigilant now about backing up. So join me on a stress-free journey to coping with stress.

Understanding Stress

What actually is stress? Stress is defined as a reaction to a physical, mental or emotional stimulus that upsets the body's natural balance – so it can range from racing to catch a plane, to trying to solve a logistical problem, to dealing with a relationship breakdown, laptop failure, even a bad haircut.

Stress is a survival mechanism – it evolved when our lives were in some ways simpler, more black and white, when it was a case of life or death; hunted or the hunter. We have evolved to do so many things now, but funnily enough our bodies haven't caught up – they still think we are roaming the savannah millions of years ago and our instincts are still geared to surviving a day on the African plains as opposed to negotiating a busy high street or coping with the politics of office life.

The Science of Stress

If you know why something is happening, then you are more likely to be able to deal with it. You have two adrenal glands which sit on top of each kidney. When instructed by your brain, they produce hormones to deal with stress. The adrenals consist of two parts – the outer larger part is the adrenal cortex and the smaller inner part is the adrenal medulla. When the brain signals that there is a threat to your status quo – a traffic warden is approaching your parked car, for example – the adrenal medulla releases the hormone adrenalin and the neurotransmitter noradrenalin into your bloodstream. This is so you are equipped for 'fight-or-flight', either run away or stand your ground and fight.

- Your pulse rate and your blood pressure go up, because your heart is beating faster so more blood can be pumped to your muscles for running away, and to your brain also for quick thinking.
- Blood is diverted away from the intestine, a lack of blood which causes a sensation of 'butterflies' in the stomach.
- Blood is also diverted away from your reproductive organs – no time for flirting and reproducing – and towards your

brain, muscles and skin, for rapid cooling on exertion, so you might feel your hands and feet getting cold.

- Your sweat glands are switched on, ready to cool your body during sudden exercise.
- Your muscles tense ready for action – you stiffen and tremble with fear and your voice might even become high-pitched and shaky.
- Your breathing rate goes up and your airways widen to bring extra oxygen into your body – you may breathe in suddenly and deeply, described as catching your breath.
- Your sugar levels increase as the body's stores are raised to provide instant energy for extra power, strength and speed.
- Your pupils dilate to improve your field of vision – your eyes can literally widen with fear.
- Chemicals are released into your blood which will make it clot more easily, and cause damaged blood vessels to constrict to reduce bleeding from potential wounds.

All this is triggered because you panicked when you saw a man with a bright yellow bib and a digital camera on the opposite side of the street! When the cause of the stress is short lived, it is known as acute stress.

But if it's not traffic wardens, it could be coping with other pedestrians, juggling jobs, making a shopping decision, difficult bosses, coping with good and bad relationships, emails, mobile phones, diaries – all things that make immediate demands on you – your body reacts the same. The adrenals are stimulated to release adrenalin, but as soon as you deal with one stress – the traffic warden, say – then another cause of stress pops up; your mobile rings, then there is a text, so your adrenals release another hormone, cortisol.

Cortisol's role is to regulate your metabolism and your

resistance to stress. Cortisol curbs functions that are not needed in a fight-or-flight situation. It alters immune system responses and suppresses the digestive system, the reproductive system and growth processes. But if you are under continual or chronic stress, then cortisol rather than controlling the problem, becomes itself a problem.

Too much cortisol in the bloodstream can have an adverse effect:

- Weight gain: cortisol causes insulin resistance and as a result excess cortisol can cause weight gain and slow down the metabolism. Also people experiencing chronic stress tend to crave more fatty, salty and sugary foods, thanks to the circulating cortisol which programs you into thinking you need a reward after all your 'exertions'. Higher levels of stress are linked to greater levels of abdominal fat.

- Over a longer time, insulin resistance sets in and your pancreas will struggle to produce enough insulin, which is why stress can lead to type II diabetes.

- You might feel weakness and pain in your muscles, as they can't take up glucose efficiently due to insulin resistance from cortisol.

- Digestion is impaired so you are less able to absorb nutrients which may make you more vulnerable to food allergies.

- Continual activation of stress hormones can raise your heart rate and increase your blood pressure and cholesterol levels.

- Lowered immunity – cortisol suppresses the immune system. There is no point building up white blood cells and protein for repair if you are going to be 'history' any minute.

- Lack of sex drive – the adrenal glands are so busy producing cortisol and adrenalin for stress, they are diverted from making sex hormone. The enzyme for making oestrogen is also depleted.

- Osteoporosis – the adrenal glands are diverted from making the enzyme which makes sex hormones which are involved in bone density.
- Feelings of depression, gloom and anxiety – certain by-products of cortisol act as sedatives, which can contribute to an overall feeling of depression.
- Sleeplessness. Cortisol follows circadian rhythms peaking at 8am and declining at night time. The function of cortisol is to make the body alert and aroused, so if cortisol levels are high at night, it is hard to sleep.
- Continual activation of stress hormones may alter the operation and structure of brain cells that are critical for memory formation and function.

If you continually subject your body to stressful situations, the adrenals get over-stimulated, so you feel the need to constantly stimulate them by drinking more coffee or eating more sweet things – until they give up and cortisol levels fall, leaving you unable to do anything. This is known as chronic fatigue syndrome. This is your body's last cry: 'stop, enough!'

But there is no need to get to this stage. Stressful events are a fact of life, but you can take steps to manage the impact these events have on you. You can learn to identify what stresses you out, how to take control of some stress-inducing circumstances, and how to take care of yourself physically and emotionally when you face events you can't control. Strategies include healthy eating, exercise, relaxation techniques and socialising with friends and family.

Stress Is Not All Bad

An appropriate stress response is a healthy and necessary part of life – otherwise life would be very boring. The adrenal medulla also releases norepinephrine, or noradrenalin, one of your principal excitatory neurotransmitters. Norepinephrine is needed to create new memories. It can improve your mood, encourage creative thinking and increase motivation. That is why you might read a thriller, go to a scary movie, take up bungee jumping . . . It is still good to have a bit of stress in your life – so don't get too horizontal.

Eat to Beat Stress

Balance Blood Sugar

It is stressful for the body to have fluctuations in blood sugar as the pancreas has to produce more insulin to transport glucose in and out of body cells. Cortisol causes more sugar to be converted from stored glycogen so you have more energy, but it also causes you to crave fast-release energy foods such as chocolate or crisps. But sadly most of our perceived stresses do not require a huge calorie input which will then have to be burned off. Dieting and fasting add to dietary stress by placing extra demands on the system to maintain blood sugar balance, so don't try any radical food changes if you are going through a stressful time of life. Eat little and often and combine a complex carbohydrate with a protein – see introduction for more details on blood sugar management.

B Vitamins

The B vitamins support the entire nervous system and some of the adrenal glands. They are also essential for energy production and provide support to the immune system (which suffers greatly under chronic stress). The B vitamins also help maintain regular blood sugar levels, which may become irregular due to stress. Foods which contain B vitamins include broccoli, wholegrains, lentils, salmon, corn, nuts, sunflower seeds, eggs and citrus fruit.

Vitamin C
Vitamin C is a key nutrient in boosting the immune system, which is also affected by stress. Vitamin C is a great help in stressful situations. It may reduce blood pressure as well as reduce the actual symptoms of stress as it has the ability to lower cortisol levels. Foods which contain vitamin C include citrus fruits, green leafy vegetables, tomatoes, broccoli, mango, and red and green bell peppers.

Protein
Amino acids are the building blocks of protein (which is found in every cell of the body). They support brain function, especially the neurotransmitters which can have a dramatic impact on mood and behaviour. Because of this, amino acids can help relieve symptoms of stress. Amino acids are found in eggs, meat, fish and pulses and grains. So if under stress, it is important to eat some protein, especially with carbohydrate in order to manage blood sugar.

Exercise
One of the best stress-busting tactics is to do some kind of physical exercise. This uses up all the stress hormones which are circulating. Exercise reduces stress through boosting circulation and the flow of lymph fluid. It also elevates your mood, so it is good to do some exercise which raises the heart

rate every day. When you finish exercising, your body will naturally switch off the cortisol and adrenalin as it thinks fight-or-flight is over.

Avoid competitive exercise, which can only aggravate a stressful situation – walking, jogging and relaxing cycling as opposed to full on cycling are good ways to de-stress. Yoga and Pilates also count as exercise; gentle exercise can have far more benefits than pounding the treadmill relentlessly.

Say No to . . .

Caffeine: be wary of too much coffee, tea, fizzy drinks and chocolate, as they are all stimulants. Not only does caffeine put a strain on your body by producing an adrenalin effect – increased heartbeat, etc. – it can also lead to increased levels of cortisol in the blood. Your body thinks it is preparing for a fight/flight response rather than relaxing with a latte and the newspaper, so your body produces cortisol to try and balance the effects of this extra 'adrenalin'. As little as two cups of coffee a day can cause nervousness, insomnia and headaches. Caffeine also lowers the thresholds for stress reactions, so you are more likely to interpret an event as stressful if you drink too much caffeine. Caffeine also uses up your reserves of the B vitamins, which are important in coping with stress, while the acidity of caffeine may affect the lining of your intestinal tract and cause inflammation.

> Two cups of coffee a day can cause nervousness, insomnia and headaches

Sugar: fast-release sugar upsets your blood sugar balance and causes increased levels of cortisol, which makes you crave more sugar, then more cortisol is produced in response to high sugar levels in the bloodstream. Excess sugar depletes vitamins and minerals, especially B vitamins which are essential for the normal functioning of your nervous system, so cut back on typical reward foods such as biscuits, cakes and processed foods.

Alcohol: booze is also high in sugar and will raise your blood sugar levels. It also depletes your body's B vitamins, and can disrupt sleep and impair your judgment and thought processes.

Nicotine: this mimics adrenalin and also depletes vitamin C. Drugs such as cocaine, barbiturates, anti-depressants, amphetamines, and marijuana deprive the body of nutrients in general, especially the B vitamins.

It's All in the Mind

You have three options when confronted with a potentially stressful situation:

- You can react.
- You can choose not to react.
- You can allow yourself to be the victim of circumstances and not do anything about the stressful situation. This is the worst situation, because once you are in this mode, your energy plummets and you are locked into a deep hole of anger and frustration because you did not choose the first two options.

Sometimes if are under too much chronic stress then you need more than positive thinking and you should seek professional help.

To make the most of your time – and avoid getting stressed by too many things:

- Learn to prioritise; decide what is an important task to do in a day – you will feel so empowered if you manage just one task.
- Make lists.
- Introduce a routine which you can control.
- Start one project and finish it before you take on another.
- Make sure you have one relaxing fifteen to twenty minute time-out treat a day – a walk in the park, listening to relaxing music, or call a friend.
- Socially, don't say yes to everything; think if you really want to do it.
- Reduce the number of hours you spend at work.
- Start an enjoyable exercise – rest your mind.
- Try relaxing techniques – things you think you don't have time for such as yoga, Pilates; have a massage.
- Set aside time to eat meals.
- Don't watch TV or read while you are eating. Try to spend fifteen to twenty minutes enjoying your food – so all the blood can be devoted to digestion. Enjoy the peace or put on some music that relaxes you or make time to eat with a friend.
- Another way to gain strength from a situation is to look back on past situations in which you did manage to overcome stress and draw strength from that.

First thing, when you wake up in the morning, decide how you want your day to go; think about it and view it positively. Before I started my cycle ride from Hong Kong to Sydney, a fellow cyclist gave me some advice – you have to be the one that smiles first. I found that advice invaluable. Although it took energy to decide to smile first, to be friendly, even when I wasn't in a good mood; to answer where I was going for the hundredth time in an hour, I was repaid many times over. I noticed on days when I woke up in a bad mood or decided I couldn't be bothered, then people were not so nice to me; things went wrong and overall I did not have such a good day. The power of positive thinking is an amazing thing.

Recipes

Cooking can be very therapeutic; who needs a stress ball when you have two onions on which to take out your frustrations? Treat yourself and don't have a slice of toast at the end of a hard day – invite 'yourself' to dinner and make a non-stressful meal from the recipes here, even if it's just lentil soup. All the recipes are easy to shop for and easy to cook – there are no hard-to-find ingredients, no stress-inducing last-minute marinating or sauces that could curdle.

Another good way to cope with stress is to socialise. Invite friends over for a meal, you don't need to make it too complicated; Spanish omelette and green salad is a good communal meal with a bottle of Spanish red (one glass won't undo all the good you've eaten) and finish with a pot of fresh mint tea and a few squares of dark chocolate. Make time to write a shopping list and allow time to shop and chop, then time to relax and eat. You will feel all the better for it the next day.

Always have breakfast – start off the day with a complex carbohydrate, good fat and protein and you will have stable blood sugar levels to help you cope with whatever the day throws at you. Don't allow yourself to say 'I am too busy, too stressed for breakfast': this is your first line of attack against stress. Eat before you make for the front door. Rye bread toasted with a nut butter is a great carbohydrate/protein/fat start to the day. Save time and make a smoothie the night before and drink it en route, or take the homemade granola in a box and eat on the move, if you have to. Eating on the run is not ideal, but it is better than not eating at all.

Bircher Muesli

This muesli is always worth getting up for. I first discovered it on a press trip in Bangkok when we were due to take the morning flight to Hong Kong. The Mandarin Oriental hotel's outdoor buffet table was groaning with fruit, pastries, noodles, eggs and cereals, but it was the Swiss-inspired Bircher muesli that I fell in love with. Oats soaked in apple juice and cream plus nuts, seeds and fresh fruits – I couldn't get enough of it, I went back for bowl after bowl.

Because of my greed, we were late setting off for the airport and Bangkok is notorious for traffic jams . . . Five of us in a taxi, in a traffic jam and the next flight was not for another week. I would not like to live through that again – there are only so many times you can say you're sorry.

However, the magnesium in the huge amount of oats I had consumed was helping to calm me and I had the benefit of loads of slow-release sugar. But that wasn't helping my fellow passengers. We did catch our flight – just.

Bircher muesli is named for its inventor, Dr Bircher-Benner, a Swiss physician and a pioneer in nutrition research who also ran a popular health clinic in Zurich during the 1890s. Developed for patients whose treatment included a diet rich in fresh fruits and vegetables, Bircher-Benner's original oat mix was soaked in condensed milk (a tuberculosis outbreak had left the public wary of fresh milk), lemon juice and grated apple.

Compared with dry oats, soaked oats are easier to digest –

but I wouldn't recommend condensed milk as it is very high in sugar! Oat products have been shown to help lower high blood cholesterol levels so oats along with their low GI properties are an excellent way to start a stress-free day.

Serves 4

Ingredients

200g jumbo porridge oats
75g raisins
300ml water or apple juice
juice of 1 lemon
2 apples, washed
125ml natural yoghurt

25g flaked almonds, toasted
150g chopped pears, mashed
   banana or fresh berries
2–4 tablespoons clear honey
sunflower and pumpkin seeds
   (optional)

Method

Prepare the oats the night before, then you can wake and go.

Place the oats and raisins in a bowl and pour over the cold water/apple juice and the lemon juice. Leave in the fridge for at least 2 hours or overnight.

Just before you are ready to eat, grate the apple and stir into the soaked oat mix. Stir in the yoghurt, almonds, fresh fruit and honey then serve sprinkled with sunflower and pumpkin seeds if you want.

The soaked oat mix will keep in the fridge for a couple of days, just add the remaining ingredients on the morning you wish to eat.

B vitamins are essential for the conversion of food into energy, and also stimulate cell growth and produce antibodies which help fight infection. Vitamin B5 (panothenic acid) is often called the anti-stress vitamin, as it helps to support the adrenal glands and improves coping mechanisms. B5 is found in wholegrains such as oats, barley, brown rice, nuts, mushrooms, eggs and avocados. B vitamins work best when you eat the whole range, so if you are taking supplements do not isolate a B vitamin, but take a complex.

Laid-back Rocky Granola Crunch

I discovered granola (crunchy oat-based breakfast cereal) when I was in Canada, where it is very popular. It's packed with B vitamins for energy and slow-release energy and magnesium from the oats. I found Canadians to be very relaxed and laid-back – could this be due to all the granola they're eating?

You can buy granola in bar form and as breakfast cereal but it is far nicer to make your own. Make up your granola ahead and you'll have a great store-cupboard source of slow-release energy. It does contain sugar, but this is balanced by the oats, nuts and seeds.

I got this recipe from Carol who manages Mount Engadine lodge, a delightful wooden chalet-style hotel in the heart of the Rockies in Alberta. The fishing scene from *Brokeback Mountain* was shot nearby and, apparently, the film's director Ang Lee and star Heath Ledger would hang out at the hotel with a few beers after filming.

After a few bowlfuls of Carol's granola for breakfast I felt wonderful and was ready for a relaxing day hiking in the hills.

Makes about 20 portions of granola

Ingredients

450g pecan nuts
220g sunflower seeds
200g walnuts
600g rolled oats
½ teaspoon salt
3 teaspoons cinnamon
1 teaspoon ground cloves

1½ teaspoons whole nutmeg, grated
250ml honey
300ml maple syrup
200ml vegetable oil
300g dried cranberries
200g raisins

Method

Preheat the oven to 130°C/250°F/Gas 1.

Toast the pecans, seeds and walnuts in a thick-bottomed pan over a low heat till just colouring. Remove from the heat and mix in the oats, salt, cinnamon, cloves and nutmeg.

In another pan, warm the honey, maple syrup and oil then tip in the spicy oat mixture and mix.

Spread on a greased baking sheet and bake for about 1 hour, checking and stirring the mixture every 15 minutes. Bake till just golden brown. Allow to cool then break up any clumps and mix in the cranberries and raisins.

Serve with soya milk or fruit juice or take as a snack to nibble during the day and keep your blood sugar steady. Stores in an airtight jar for up to 1 month.

Breakfast Millet with Almonds and Apricots

Millet is a great source of vitamin B5, iron and also protein. It takes longer to cook than porridge oats, but is a nice alternative as it is lighter in texture – when cooked the tiny golden seeds go all fluffy. It is lovely eaten on a summer's morning – sun streaming into the kitchen – with some fresh fruit and yoghurt.

Makes 1 large or 2 small portions

Ingredients

50g millet

200ml water

6 dried apricots (dark orange unsulphured ones are best), chopped

salt to taste

30g flaked almonds

yoghurt to moisten (optional)

honey to sweeten (optional)

pumpkin seeds (optional)

Method

Rinse and drain the millet then add to the water and simmer in a pan with the apricots for about 10 minutes or till the water has been absorbed. Add salt to taste and stir in the almonds.

Serve with a little yoghurt to moisten along with a dollop of honey and pumpkin seeds.

Mushroom and Barley Risotto

This risotto is a warming, comforting dish. Mushrooms and barley are both rich in restorative B5 vitamins.

Serves 2

Ingredients

knob of butter
1 onion, chopped
200g pearl or pot barley
pinch of dried thyme
1 bay leaf

1 litre chicken stock
1 tablespoon olive oil
400g standard mushrooms, sliced
2 cloves garlic, chopped
bunch of fresh parsley, chopped

Method

Melt the butter in a large, deep pan. Add the onion and cook till soft. Add the barley, thyme, bay leaf and 500ml of hot stock. Bring to the boil then reduce the heat and simmer till most of the stock has been absorbed, which should take about 10 minutes. Add the rest of the stock, a ladleful at a time, stirring between each. Wait for each addition to become absorbed before adding the next.

Meanwhile, heat the olive oil in a large frying pan and sauté the mushrooms until tender. Add the garlic, and cook for a couple of minutes more.

Finally, stir in the barley mixture and parsley and serve.

Lentil Soup with a Kick

Lentils are a good source of vitamin B and this recipe gives them a spicy kick.

To transform the soup into a delicious stew, use less stock and swap 150g lentils for 150g of Indian split peas.

Serves 4

Ingredients

Lentil Soup

2 tablespoons olive oil
1 onion, finely chopped
3 cloves garlic, very finely
   chopped
2 teaspoons each of ground
   cumin and cumin seeds

1 teaspoon each of ground
   coriander and coriander
   seeds
300g red lentils
400g can chopped tomatoes
1 litre chicken stock

Sweet and Spicy Fried Onions

1 tablespoon olive oil
2 onions, very finely sliced
1 teaspoon ground cinnamon
2 teaspoons soft brown sugar
1 medium red chilli, deseeded
   and finely chopped

juice of ½ lemon
Greek yoghurt and parsley to
   garnish (optional)

Method

In a large pan, heat the olive oil and cook the onion till soft. Add the garlic, spices and cook for a couple of minutes to release the flavours then stir in the rest of the ingredients. Add the hot stock and simmer for about 30 minutes or till the lentils have completely broken down.

To make the spicy topping, heat the olive oil in a frying pan till very hot then add the onions and fry till golden. Add the cinnamon, sugar and chilli. Once the sugar is no longer granular, add the lemon juice. Top the soup with sweet, spicy onions and serve garnished with yoghurt and parsley.

Chicken, Avocado and Mango Salad with Hazelnut Honey Dressing

Magnesium and calcium are essential for optimum nerve function and leafy greens, such as the watercress used in this recipe, are a good source of both. The vivid orange mango and green, creamy avocado in this colourful salad are a lovely way to boost your vitamin C and antioxidant intake as well as its protein-packed, calcium-rich nuts.

For a quicker-to-make salad use smoked chicken breast – you don't need to cook the chicken and its smokiness perfectly complements the mango and avocado.

Serves 4

Ingredients

Chicken, Avocado and Mango Salad

750ml chicken stock
juice of 1 lime
4 chicken breasts
1 ripe avocado

1 ripe mango or 100g frozen mango
chunks, defrosted
100g watercress

Hazelnut Honey Dressing

3 tablespoons sunflower oil

3 tablespoons sesame oil

finely grated rind and juice
  of 1 lime

3 tablespoons clear honey

3 tablespoons sodium reduced
  soy sauce

100g hazelnuts, toasted and
  roughly chopped

Method

Put the stock and lime juice in a saucepan, add the chicken breasts and poach for about 20 minutes or till the chicken is cooked through. To check the chicken is cooked, slide a knife into the centre of the breast, ease the meat apart and you should see no trace of pink.

Remove the chicken from the pan with a slotted spoon, allow to cool on a plate then cut into bite-sized pieces.

Cut the avocado and the mango in half then stone, peel and finely slice both.

In a serving bowl, toss together the avocado, mango, chicken and watercress.

To make the hazelnut honey dressing, put all the ingredients except the hazelnuts into a bowl and whisk to mix, then stir in the hazelnuts.

Pour the dressing over the salad and toss lightly so that all the salad ingredients are well coated.

Sweet Potato Omelette

Eggs are a great source of protein and all the B vitamins. There is something very comforting about eggs and this big Spanish-style omelette (tortilla) is great for slicing and sharing.

Serve with a leafy green salad sprinkled with pumpkin seeds.

Serves 2

Ingredients

300g sweet potatoes, scrubbed and peeled
1 large Spanish onion
3 tablespoons olive oil

6 eggs
sea salt and freshly ground black pepper
flat leaf parsley to garnish

Method

You will need a large, non-stick frying pan with a lid plus a plate at least the same diameter as the pan.

Thinly slice the potatoes and onion into half rings. Heat 2 tablespoons of the oil in the frying pan, add the potatoes and onion and cook, lid on over a low heat, stirring occasionally, till the potatoes are cooked through (about 25 minutes). Remove from the heat and allow to cool a little.

In a large bowl, beat the eggs. To the beaten eggs, gently add the potato and onion slices and season with salt and pepper.

Heat the remaining oil in the frying pan, tip in the egg and potato mixture in an even layer and cook very slowly for about 10 minutes, or till the tortilla sets.

To brown the top of the tortilla, place a large plate, upside down, over the pan. Now invert the pan so that the tortilla sits, cooked side up, on the plate. Slide the tortilla, uncooked side down, back into the pan and allow to brown for a couple of minutes.

Finally, turn the tortilla out on to the plate again, cut into wedges and serve hot or cold garnished with lots of flat leaf parsley.

Easy Peasy Spicy Pork Skewers

These are so easy to make and they are an easy – and delicious – way to access protein.

I made them during a food demonstration in a marquee in Glasgow's George Square. My only stress was when my oven glove caught fire on the hot grill but, luckily, the audience assumed the flame was part of the barbeque experience.

Serve on a bed of brown rice or with a bean salad. You can replace the pork with chicken or fish cut into small pieces.

Serves 4–6 as a starter

Ingredients

400g pork tenderloin
2 garlic cloves, crushed
40g ginger, peeled and chopped
1 red chilli, deseeded and sliced
sea salt and freshly ground
     black pepper

2 limes: 1 lime juiced, 1 lime
     cut in thin wedges
6 bamboo skewers, soaked in
     water for 30 minutes to
     prevent them burning

Method

Cut the pork into thin strips.

Mix together the garlic, ginger, chilli, salt, pepper and lime juice in a shallow dish, add the pork, and leave to marinate in the fridge for at least 30 minutes. Thread the meat on to skewers and cook under a red-hot grill for 5–10 minutes, turning once. Serve with lime wedges on the side.

Smoked Mackerel Dip

Oily fish is good when you're feeling stressed as it can help balance blood sugar and mood swings. The omega 3s in oily fish improve your body's ability to respond to insulin so are good for blood sugar balance.

It can be hard to incorporate oily fish into your diet as often as the recommended three times a week but this versatile smoked mackerel recipe should help. Serve it as a dip with carrot and celery sticks, use it as a sandwich filling, in salads or even add it as a sauce to pasta – plenty of ways to deliver those essential omega 3s.

Serves 2–3

Ingredients

100g smoked mackerel fillets
150g thick, Greek natural
  yoghurt

2 tablespoons lemon juice
freshly ground black pepper
  to season

Method

Remove the most prominent bones from the mackerel and whizz in a blender together with the yoghurt and lemon juice. Season with pepper and enjoy.

Lemon and Thyme Roasted Cod

Cod is a good source of protein – essential for tissue repair – and it is also rich in magnesium and calcium, which help you relax. This easy-to-cook recipe is given real zing by the lemon and capers. Serve with wilted greens or a tomato salad.

Serves 4

Ingredients

4 fresh or frozen cod fillets, each weighing 125g

10 pitted green olives

2 tablespoons capers

zest and juice of 1 lemon

1 tablespoon olive oil

a few sprigs of fresh thyme

Method

Preheat the oven to 180°C/350°F/Gas 4.

Roughly chop the olives and capers, transfer to a small bowl and add the lemon zest, juice and olive oil. Tear off a few thyme leaves, add to the bowl and mix everything together.

Lay the cod in an oiled roasting tin and spoon over the lemon and thyme mix.

Cover the tin with foil and roast for 15–20 minutes until the fish is cooked through and flakes easily.

Gooey Dark Chocolate Raspberry Almond Cakes

Almonds are a good source of calming magnesium and this is a nice, comforting pudding.

Be brave and remove the cakes from the oven when they still look 'wobbly' – you're aiming for gooey centres of molten chocolate and hot raspberry.

Egg yolks are a good source of nervous system-friendly vitamin B so use the leftover yolks here in scrambled egg or in *Sweet Potato Omelette*, see page 153.

Serves 6

Ingredients

80g unsalted butter	75g icing sugar
160g dark chocolate	150g ground almonds
2 egg whites, beaten	6 frozen raspberries
50g self raising flour	

Method

Preheat the oven to 150°C/300°F/Gas 2. You will need 6 large muffin cases.

Melt the butter and the chocolate, slowly, in a bowl over a pan of hot water (don't let the base of the bowl touch the water) and allow to cool.

Beat the egg whites to stiff peaks then gently fold in the flour, icing sugar and almonds. Then gently stir into the butter and chocolate mixture.

Spoon half the mixture into muffin cases, half-filling each case. Place a raspberry in the centre of each case then top with remaining mixture.

Bake for 20 minutes – the cakes should feel soft to the touch. Allow to rest for 5 minutes before eating.

Anti-stress Checklist

- Maintain blood sugar balance by eating regular meals with some protein, good fat and complex carbohydrate at each meal.
- Cut right back on caffeine as it mimics adrenalin.
- Limit alcohol to no more than seven units a week.
- Exercise at least three times a week for twenty to thirty minutes.
- Stress management is the key, not stress elimination, so decide each day you won't get stressed.
- Make sure you do something each day that gives you pure pleasure.

Have a Nice Stress-free Day!

Breakfast: prepare granola or bircher muesli the night before, so you can rise, shine and go. Oats are a good source of slow-release energy, so keep sugar levels even which is an antidote to stress. Oats are rich in calming magnesium.

Snack: five almonds – calming as they also contain magnesium.

Lunch: hot or cold sweet potato omelette (made the day before and taken into work), rich in stress-beating vitamin B5 eggs, with green salad.

Snack: smoked mackerel dip with oatcakes – oily fish helps balance hormones and oatcakes for magnesium and energy.

Evening meal: chicken, mango and avocado salad – lots of vitamin C and antioxidants; there's calcium in the watercress and magnesium in the hazelnuts, so this is a nice salad to have in the evening as the calcium/magnesium combo is very relaxing.

Water: keep hydrated so 1.5 litres and more if hot and exercising.

Exercise: go for a thirty-minute walk or take a Pilates class – less stressful than yoga which can be intimidating and stressful if you can't bend as much as everyone else.

Bonuses: as well as feeling calmer and less anxious, you will have more energy; wounds will heal quicker and you can benefit from lower cholesterol, clear skin and strong hair.

Your Beautiful Skin – and Hair and Nails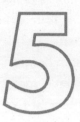

I was flicking through a women's magazine looking for recipe ideas and general life-improving advice, as you do, when I started noticing the skin advertisements promoting products which can 'target wrinkles', 'help to protect against environmental irritants', promote a 'younger-looking you', promise 'advanced anti-ageing sun protection' and 'beauty enhancing pigments that can give your skin a subtle glow'. Then I thought I could offer you similar benefits with *Eat Well with Nell* and at a fraction of the cost – though avocados ripening on the dressing room table or jars of oatmeal and almond oil in the bathroom cabinet can't quite compare with beautifully packaged tubes and bottles. But stick with me, we can work together on this; I am not saying give up on the lotions and potions, but first think about your diet. No skin cream, however expensive, can work wonders on a skin ravaged by junk food, biscuits, cakes, alcohol, smoking and sun. Try and improve your diet and lifestyle; you may not need so many packaged beauty products, and the bonus is you will have glowing, healthy, smooth skin – and lovely strong hair and nails. I'll expand on hair and nails at the end of the chapter.

Your skin is your body's largest organ and your vitality, health and in fact your emotional state are all mirrored in your skin. Many of my clients think healthy skin belongs in the hands of the beautician rather than the nutritionist and are surprised if I ask them about theirs – even though many beauty creams boast of containing vitamins A, C and E. Nutrition can also play a huge part in helping people with specific skin complaints such as acne, cellulite, eczema and psoriasis – again areas where people may not resort to food as their first ally.

Your Skin

Your skin is not only your largest organ but it does so much for you. Foremost, it protects your internal systems. It is the first line of defence against harmful external factors such as viruses, bacteria, chemicals and sunlight from which it can make vitamin D. Your skin is crucial for regulating body temperature through sweating and when you are hot, the blood vessels in your skin dilate, so more blood can get to the surface to cool you down. When you are cold, the vessels contract to conserve body heat.

Your skin is sensitive and warns you against harm by registering physical pain such as heat, cold and sharp things. It allows sweat and oil to be excreted as perspiration. I remember discovering baked garlic for the first time and I loved spreading the rich pungent caramelly paste which oozed from the baked clove onto bread – only to discover a few hours later in a very hot Hong Kong bar, that everyone else was acutely aware of my new found love. Don't let me put you off baked garlic and all its nutritional benefits – I did eat a lot and it was very hot . . .

The skin acts as a two-way system of exchange, just as it can excrete, it can also absorb substances such as fat-soluble vitamins, nicotine patches and steroids.

Your skin consists of three layers – the outermost layer, the epidermis; the middle supporting layer, the dermis, and an inner subcutaneous layer. The epidermis is made up of four types of cells, mainly keratinocytes which are renewed every two to four weeks. It is the keratinocytes which give your skin its waterproof coating. They are the cells which turn brown when the melanocytes are stimulated by sunlight to produce the pigment melanin to protect the skin cells from UV light.

The dermis is the next layer down, and is where all the beauty buzzwords are found; the dermis is made up of proteins called collagen and elastin – they form the skin's supporting structure and help to act as a shock absorber. Collagen is the largest part of the skin's support structure, a tightly organised mesh of fibres which inevitably break down over time. Collagen fibres contain elastin. Elastin acts like an elastic band and springs the skin back into shape. Elastin is damaged by repeated exposure to the sun, especially UV waves, and also by inflammation in the skin. Once damaged, elastin becomes dry and brittle which leads to wrinkles and sagging. Wrinkles are a sign that the skin is losing some of its elasticity but through diet and lifestyle you can delay the process. The dermis also helps to maintain the supply of nutrients, water and electrolytes to the epidermis. Working backwards, fibroblasts are cells in the dermis which produce the proteins collagen and elastin – retin A beauty creams stimulate their production. The dermis also contains hair follicles and sweat glands. Cells are produced in the dermis then work their way up to the epidermis; it is the dermis that absorbs moisturisers.

Moisturisers

Your skin has its own built-in moisturiser – your sweat. Sweat acts as an acidic barrier and the sebum produced by the sebaceous glands keeps moisture in. Be careful not to over-moisturise as you may end up sealing the pores and preventing your skin from breathing. Your neck has no sebaceous glands and therefore no natural oils, so it will always be grateful for some moisturiser. Likewise the delicate skin under your eyes which has very few sebaceous glands.

Moisturisers work by adding water to the skin cells, plumping them up for only about twelve hours. It is best to apply a moisturiser after showering, when your skin is still wet, and the oils in the moisturiser will trap the moisture on your skin. Look at the list of ingredients on bought moisturisers and the first ingredient from the most expensive to the supermarket special will be water or, if they are going down the more sophisticated route, aqua. A cheap, cheerful and effective moisturiser is nut or seed oil which is rich in vitamin E; put a tiny amount of, say, almond oil on your palm and add a drop of warm water, rub your palms together and apply to your skin after cleansing.

The third layer of your skin is the subcutaneous layer. This is the deepest and is mainly made up of fat – fat which plumps up wrinkles and prevents a scrawny look. This layer of fat is criss-crossed by blood vessels, nerve fibres and fibrous cells. It is vital for normal functioning of your skin. You have more subcutaneous fat over the thighs, tummy and buttocks than on your eyelids.

Healthy Beautiful Skin Needs:

Water Water, which you need both inside and out! Plump up the cells from within by drinking water. The recommended amount of water you should drink per day is about one and a half litres, but it also depends on how much fruit and vegetables you eat – they contain water – or how much coffee you drink, which is a diuretic which causes you to lose water. Drink until your urine is pale yellow; if darker, then you need to take in more water. Remember herbal teas count! And on the outside, use vegetable or seed oils or your favourite moisturiser straight after showering, without drying, to trap moisture on your skin.

Antioxidants Antioxidants, which are nutrients that protect your body from damage by free radicals, the unstable molecules in your body that undermine your long-term health. In humans, the most common form of free radicals is the oxygen-free radical. This is produced when oxygen is used in normal cell processes such as respiration and energy production and is increased by exposure to pollution, radiation, junk food, alcohol and smoking. In the oxidation process, sometimes an oxygen molecule loses one of its electrons from its outer shell. This turns it into a free radical so it is forced to whizz about trying to steal an electron from another stable oxygen molecule to make itself stable. An antioxidant sacrifices itself by giving up its electron to make the oxygen molecule stable again. Too many unstable electrons, i.e. free radicals, causes irreversible damage and can lead to disease. Free radicals cause cross linking between collagen fibres and encourage wrinkle formation as elasticity decreases. So forget the hips when you tuck into a cheap biscuit made with hydrogenated fats, think of your face and your collagen fibres!

Help is instantly at hand – antioxidants which are abundant in fruit and vegetables and in some grains, nuts, meat and fish – can neutralise the free oxygen radical and stop it creating havoc with its neighbouring electrons. Brightly coloured fruit and vegetables are natural sources of antioxidants, as the pigment which gives them their colour was originally designed to protect the plant. Vitamins A, C and E also have antioxidant properties – they can neutralise any free radicals in the body. Minerals found in nuts help antioxidants react with the free radicals. An amino acid, glutathione, is sometimes called the 'master antioxidant' as in addition to its own antioxidant powers, glutathione can help to recycle other antioxidants such as vitamins C and E. Glutathione can be found in fruit and vegetables, especially asparagus, avocado, walnuts, fish and meat.

Vitamin A This is responsible for the general maintenance of your skin as it is involved in creating new cells. So it is no surprise to find it in many anti-ageing creams. Vitamin A is found in high concentrations in the dermis and epidermis, as it also affects the rate of keratinisation – a deficiency of vitamin A means dry, scaly skin. Foods rich in vitamin A or retinol are animal livers and herring and mackerel and it is present as beta carotene in all red and orange fruit and vegetables such as pumpkin, tomatoes, apricots and mangoes.

Vitamin C This is required in the production of collagen – a protein which makes your skin look soft and youthful. As well as aesthetic skin maintenance, vitamin C is vital in maintaining healthy tissue, bones and teeth, as well as aiding the body's absorption of iron and helping to heal any wounds. Vitamin C is also an important antioxidant vitamin, for example it can deactivate sun-induced free radicals in the skin which, left unattended can trigger sun damage. Most fruit and vegetables contain vitamin C.

Vitamin D This is needed for regular growth of new skin cells. It may help psoriasis sufferers where cells are being over-renewed, which is why sunlight is recommended for psoriasis sufferers. Try to spend about twenty minutes outside every day to get your vitamin D from the sun, though not at midday, and fill up on oily fish, fish oils and eggs.

Vitamin E This is a fat-soluble vitamin necessary for growth of tissue; it strengthens cell membranes and improves capillary integrity. Lack of vitamin E leads to shrinkage of collagen and increased membrane fragility, i.e. wrinkles. It is also an antioxidant and it is used topically to prevent scarring. Foods rich in vitamin E are almonds, avocados, leafy greens, hazelnuts, peanut butter and sunflower seeds.

Zinc Zinc is required for building new cells, as it supports the immune system. Zinc also helps acne, wound healing, stretch marks and eczema. Zinc-rich foods are oysters, wholegrains, eggs, sesame seeds, pumpkin seeds, almonds.

Fibre Fibre helps to bind the toxins produced after digestion. Fibre also prevents constipation, i.e. the length of time fibre, toxins, waste etc. are in the intestine. If the waste products from digestion linger too long, they can be reabsorbed back into the bloodstream causing a muddy complexion. Make sure you are eating enough fruit and vegetables plus their skins, beans, wholegrains and pulses.

Protein Your body needs protein as a building block. And where your skin is concerned, collagen and elastin consist predominantly of protein. Your skin has a high turnover of cells – your epidermis is renewed every thirty to forty days. So it is important to help your skin, by making sure you have a good selection of amino acids each day. Lean meat, fish, eggs, beans and pulses should make up fifteen to twenty-five per cent of your diet. Often lack of protein first shows in the face. But a huge steak once a week won't help, as your body very annoyingly does not store amino acids, but uses what it needs and coverts the rest into sugars and fatty acids, so it is a case of a little protein and often.

EFAs Skin cells are made from Essential Fatty Acids (EFAs) which are found in vegetable oils, nuts, cereals and oily fish. They are called essential, as your body can't make them. EFAs make cell membranes more fluid and let skin produce its own fats or lipids which act as an effective barrier against water loss, making skin smooth and supple. Without these fats, your cells can't retain water which gives them their plumpness, so a low-fat diet will soon show in your skin and your skin will be hungry for even more moisturiser. EFAs also control the speed at which healthy cells are produced.

Exercise After a healthy diet, regular exercise does more for your skin than any skin cream. Exercise causes a surge of

> After a healthy diet, regular exercise does more for your skin than any skin cream

oxygen to all organs including your skin, preventing free radical damage and stimulating circulation – very important in the fight against cellulite – the lymphatic system and perspiration that triggers the production of sebum which acts as your skin's own moisturiser. Exercise also helps manage insulin and blood sugar levels, as both are damaging to the collagen in the dermis.

Sleep It's not called beauty sleep for nothing! When you sleep your body produces the highest levels of hormones which encourage the skin to heal, with the greatest benefits occurring at the end of your sleep. Lack of sleep stresses the body which can affect the tiny blood vessels round the eyes, which is why a late night can show around your eyes next morning. Also your liver does most of its detoxing from eleven at night to three in the morning, so it is vital that you let it get on with its valuable work of expelling toxins from your body.

Your Skin Doesn't Need:
Too Much Sun Sun, or ultraviolet light to be more correct, is the cause of ninety per cent of skin ageing. Sunlight is made up of ultraviolet A and ultraviolet B wavelengths – the UVA has longer wavelengths which can penetrate deeper into the skin, breaking down the support structures of collagen and elastin. These waves also damage the enzymes that protect collagen from breakdown. UVB increases risk of skin cancer, while UVA causes premature ageing. Sunburn is an inflammation which breaks down collagen and elastin fibres.

A tan is the skin's way of protecting itself against the sun's strong rays. The pigment cells which determine how deep your tan is are found in the epidermis. They are called melanocytes and produce melanin which colours the keratinocytes and which absorbs UV parts of sunlight and also mops up the free radicals that are produced by skin in response to sun exposure. Sunlight also causes the epidermis to thicken to offer more protection.

But don't avoid the sun completely. UV rays stimulate the body's calcium and phosphate balance, encouraging calcium absorption in the gut which in turn keeps bones and teeth strong. Sun is a good source of vitamin D, but you only need about twenty minutes a day – not between 10am–2pm when the sun is at its strongest. Sunscreens only filter, they don't block sunlight, so will still allow some UV to get through to make vitamin D.

Fake tan products – how they work

I know a tan isn't good for you, but I love the feeling of being brown; it makes your eyes look brighter, teeth whiter and your white jeans dazzle the way no washing powder ever can. Most dermatologists, however, will recommend a fake tan as opposed to the real thing. The active ingredient in fake tan is Dihydroxyacetone (DHA). When applied to the skin it causes a chemical reaction with the amino acids in the surface cells of the skin, producing a darkening effect. DHA does not damage skin as it only affects the outermost cells of the epidermis. The outer skin cells are already dead, and are shed as the skin renews itself, which means fake tan has to be reapplied every couple of days and why it is important to exfoliate before each application. The DHA doesn't go beyond the outer layer of skin so isn't absorbed into the body. You should always test tanning lotion on a small area of skin before using it, in case you have an allergic reaction. The more expensive the fake tan product, the higher levels of DHA, though I can't suggest a good reply when people comment on your beautiful tan and ask where you've been. The answer 'Boots' can flummox the person who posed the question.

Sugar Sugar is on the baddie list again. American dermatologist Dr Nicholas Perricone in his books *The Wrinkle Cure* and *7 Secrets to Beauty, Health and Longevity* cites sugar as a major cause of wrinkles and dull-looking skin. Sugar raises your blood sugar which triggers an instant rise in the hormone insulin responsible for returning your blood sugar level to normal. High levels of insulin cause an inflammatory response which causes damage to collagen. Plus, when you console yourself after a bad day with a bar of milk chocolate, the sugar in your bloodstream attaches itself to proteins in your skin, i.e. collagen and elastin, to form harmful new molecules called Advanced Glycation End products (rather appropriately, abbreviated to AGEs). AGEs makes the skin stiffen and inflexible. The more AGEs there are, the more damage, as they act like a domino effect. AGEs also deactivate your body's natural antioxidant enzymes, leaving you more vulnerable to sun damage which is still the main cause of skin ageing.

But before you vow to remove sugar completely from your life in search of a wrinkle-free skin, let alone slimmer waistline, bear in mind that it is practically impossible: your body needs sugar for energy. What you can do is watch out for hidden sugars which often occur in processed foods. Beware of high fructose corn syrup especially, as this type of sweetener is made by changing the sugar in cornstarch to fructose (another form of sugar) and this is thought to produce a high number of AGEs. Because these high fructose corn syrups extend the shelf life of foods, they are often found in fizzy and fruit-flavoured drinks, and packaged foods. So the easiest way to avoid excess sugar, which will dramatically raise your blood sugar, is to avoid processed foods. Turn back to the introduction for more information on balancing your blood sugar.

Smoking Smoking reduces the amount of oxygen available to all body organs including your skin by narrowing your blood vessels, so less elastin and collagen is produced. Smoking also damages the enzymes which control collagen production and encourages free radicals.

Alcohol Constant topping up of alcohol levels causes enlargement of blood vessels, the typical 'red drinker's face'. Repeated reddening leads to spider veins, and excess alcohol can also reduce absorption of key vitamins and nutrients which your skin requires. Alcohol can also cause free radicals and water loss from your cells which translates as dry skin.

Dieting Crash diets, especially before a holiday, sound so tempting, but sadly you cannot direct where your body will use up the extra fat it has squirrelled away. Fat is stored in the subcutaneous layer, but your body does not take the fat for energy from where you think it is painfully obvious it should come from – often the body takes it from the face, neck and breasts, before any impact is made on the stomach or thighs. The high-protein Atkins diet can produce a sudden loss of fat from the face when in fat-burning phase, so it can make Atkins dieters look grey and pallid.

Sudden weight gain or loss appear as stretch marks which are caused by the widening and stretching of the collagen and elastin bundles. As your skin ages, it gets less efficient at coping with sudden changes in the supporting fat, so gradual weight loss is more beneficial in terms of your skin's fat management.

Caffeine Coffee, teas and chocolate, if consumed in large quantities, can be diuretic, drawing water away from the skin and depleting your body of vital skin-enhancing moisture. Caffeine also causes blood sugar to rise, which may make you crave sweet things. Caffeine depletes vitamins, especially the B vitamins.

When Skin Goes Wrong

Your skin is a useful barometer for the overall health of the rest of your body, so a rash or spots or irritation may indicate that your body is stressed, constipated, tired or lacking vital nutrients and minerals. The best way to treat a skin complaint is to look at the possible causes and treat the whole body through diet and lifestyle.

Acne

Acne seems so cruel; it strikes in your teens, the first time in your life you are acutely conscious of your appearance, the first time you have no parental bar to junk food and at a time when your hormones are in overdrive. Acne can occur in adults, showing as spots on the chin and jaw line if stress throws hormones off balance. Hormones increase the production of oil sebum which is produced by the sebaceous glands. If the oil ducts get blocked, bacteria get trapped which manifests itself as blackheads, whiteheads and inflamed red spots. The usual triggers are hormone imbalance, stress and some medications, along with poor digestion and stress. The best way to cope with acne is:

- Drink plenty of water to flush out toxins.
- Fibre: eat lots of vegetables and moderate amounts of fruit, wholegrains and pulses. These will keep the body in an alkaline state, so less likely to suffer from inflammatory conditions. The fibre in the fruit and vegetables will also help expel toxins from the body, promoting a clearer skin.
- EFAs and zinc-rich foods such as soybeans, wholegrains, sunflower seeds and raw nuts help balance hormones and control oil production.
- Avoid junk foods and hydrogenated fats, sugar and refined foods which promote bad bowel conditions.
- Eat live yoghurt as it can replenish healthy gut flora. You can also apply yoghurt direct to the skin as the acids, lipids and enzymes may remove dead skin cells and prevent blackheads. Apply with cotton wool and remove with warm water.
- Dairy or other food allergies can be a trigger so try eliminating suspect foods for one month.

> " The best way to try and reduce the appearance of cellulite is through stimulating your circulation "

Cellulite

Cellulite is an annoying fact of life and is the result of toxins dumped in fat cells which cause a dimpled effect mainly on the back of your legs where fat is stored. The best way to try and reduce the appearance of cellulite is through stimulating your circulation. This is why, up to a point, cellulite creams work. By rubbing in a cream you help shift the toxins which cause cellulite. Food wise:

- Cut back on saturated fats, red meat and dairy.
- Drink more water to flush out toxins.
- Eat more fruit and vegetables with skins on.
- Increase soluble fibre such as oats to remove toxins.
- Exercise will also stimulate circulation.

Eczema

Eczema is common in children and is often linked to asthma and hay fever. It manifests itself as red scaly skin or a dry patchy rash which weeps. Diet is a trigger as well as perfumes, houseplants, stress and food additives.

Try to:

- Avoid key food allergens: eggs, peanuts, dairy, fish, soy, citrus and wheat. Cut out one at a time to see which is the main trigger.
- Increase essential fatty acids in diet, so add oily fish, seeds, avocados or an EFA supplement.

- Zinc-rich foods are good for boosting the immune system.
- Correct any possible imbalance of gut flora, so try probiotics as a supplement or yoghurt if not affected by dairy.
- Apply to skin: primrose oil to reduce roughness and almond oil can prevent dryness and itching.

Psoriasis

Psoriasis is white scales on red inflamed patches on the body. It can run in families. It is caused by the cells on the outer layer of the skin never fully maturing; instead they keep replicating every eight days as opposed to every twenty-eight days leaving red flaky patches which turn silver. It is not contagious. Stress is often a reason, so turn back to stress chapter.

Food wise:

- Psoriasis flare ups can be a sign of toxicity in your body, so some sufferers adopt an almost vegan diet: no dairy, eggs, meat, fish and lots of fruit, vegetables, pulses and grains to induce an alkaline state in the body.
- Avoid citrus, dairy and coffee.
- Smoking makes flare ups more likely.
- Increase essential fatty acids in diet, but cut back on saturated fats.
- Exposure to sunlight seems to help, so make sure you have twenty minutes a day outside.

Rosacea

Rosacea is most common in women aged thirty to fifty and is caused when groups of capillaries close to the surface of the skin become dilated, resulting in blotchy red areas with small bumps. Stress and change in temperature are often blamed. See

Chapter Four on how to minimise stress through lifestyle and diet. Key food triggers in rosacea are:

- Spicy foods
- Hormonal changes
- Exercise
- Weather
- Hot liquids
- Chocolate
- Coffee
- Citrus fruits
- Alcohol

Great Hair and Beautiful Nails

Follow the advice for lovely skin and you can't help but see over a couple of months an improvement in your hair and nails, as they are basically an extension of your epidermis, the top-most layer of your skin. So if you have dry hair, because of under-active sebaceous glands, poor circulation, lack of zinc or lack of EFAs, you will probably have dry skin too. And just as greasy hair is caused by over-active sebaceous glands, you may also have greasy skin. And like your skin, age, diet, hormones, climate and seasonal changes plus stress and anxiety all have an impact on hair and nails.

Your skin sheds its top layer, the epidermis, every twenty-eight days, hair cells last for up to three to seven years, growing at a rate of 20–30mm a month until the hair falls or grows out. Every day you can lose between fifty to two hundred hairs. The hair you see is dead cells; the way to nourish your hair is through the roots, so like your skin it needs a good balanced diet rich in protein, minerals and vitamins and EFAs. The key with hair health is to have a healthy scalp so you need good circulation, in order that the blood can reach all your hair follicles for oxygen and nutrient exchange; that is why hairdressers often offer a massage when you are having your hair washed.

When It's Not a Good Hair Day:

Split Ends
Split ends are caused when the protein keratin in hair is reduced. Keratin helps the hair lock in moisture. You can't put the keratin back into the ends of your hair, but you can replicate keratin's ability to lock in moisture – try massaging coconut oil into your hair once a week. And make sure you are eating enough protein at meals to build up new skin, hair and nail cells.

Dandruff
Dandruff – white flakes and itching and redness of the scalp – is caused by an excess of dead skin cells, sometimes associated with a yeast infection or a food intolerance. A diet high in acid-forming foods – saturated fat and junk food, sugar and alcohol – will tip you over the balance, so fill up on alkaline foods: lots of wholegrains and vegetables, and seeds. Increase the amount of vitamin E in your diet to nourish your hair follicles. EFAs will also help ease any inflammation. Massage coconut oil into your scalp to moisturise hair follicles and get oxygen to them.

Greying Hair
Grey hair is caused by insufficient melanin pigment being produced in the hair follicle. It can be linked to iron deficiency and lack of B12, so vegetarians are vulnerable. Also stress,

menopause and lack of copper, zinc and folic acid can cause a reduction in melanin production. Turn back to Chapter Four on stress. B vitamins are involved in hair growth, pigment-ation and strength. You need to bump up protein and include more vitamin E in your diet – but greying hair is an age thing which is related to genetics, so there is only so much sunflower seeds and wheat germ oil can do!

Thinning and Loss of Hair

Less hair means it is growing more slowly – it is usually related to getting older as the thymus gland is slowing down. Pregnancy, menopause and stress may affect your hair. Also lack of iron can be a cause of thinning hair, so make sure you are eating enough meat, fish, seeds, wheat germ, nuts and wholegrains, along with vitamin C to aid absorption. It's worth looking at your tea and coffee drinking habits as a cup of tea within half an hour of eating an iron-rich food can reduce the nutritional value by up to eighty per cent. Try to get iron through food or as part of a multi-vitamin supplement; iron on its own, however, can unbalance the absorption of other minerals. Iodine is essential for a healthy thyroid gland – if under-active, many of your normal body functions will slow down including the growth of your hair follicles. Top up your diet with iodised salt, fish and yoghurt. More than five cups of tea will also affect iodine and iron utilisation. Women tend to lose hair from all over their scalp, whereas in men it is from the temples and the crown. Make sure your digestive system is functioning – see Chapter Seven – and make sure you have enough protein.

Nails

Your nails are mainly composed of laminated layers of keratin

– the same protein found in your top layer of skin and hair. The purpose of nails, clearly, is to protect your fingers. Your nails grow from the area under the cuticle and as the older cells become compacted, they are pushed up the nail bed by younger cells. It takes about four to six months to grow a new finger- or toenail. For healthy nails, eat as you would for the skin: EFAs, vitamin E, zinc, low-fat proteins and lots of B vitamins and water. Nails to some extent can mirror what is happening in your body, clues to poor digestion, food intolerances as well as stress and illness, so health therapists often inspect their clients' nails. Be kind to your nails, protect them from all those strong household chemicals when cleaning and washing up – wear gloves and moisturise with warm oil regularly.

Brittle, Peeling Nails This could indicate an iron deficiency, lack of vitamin A, lack of biotin, calcium and most probably lack of EFAs. Massage warm wheat germ or avocado oil into nails and cuticles before going to bed to encourage circulation and absorption of moisture.

Giddy up!

Vets sometimes recommend biotin as a supplement for horses with split hooves as biotin can improve keratin-made structures like hooves – and nails and hair! Controlled experiments were done on the famous white Lipizzaner stallions at Austria's renowned Spanish Riding School in Vienna. Horses given biotin supplements had stronger, healthier hooves which did not split, than those denied the supplement. Biotin is a water-soluble vitamin, so it can't be stored. It works with the B vitamins, breaking down fats, carbs and proteins. It is manufactured in the intestines by gut bacteria, so don't worry, you won't need to take the horse pills, as it is rare for humans to be deficient in biotin. The best sources of biotin are liver, kidney, soybeans, wholegrains, mushrooms, nuts and pulses. Alcohol, cooking, egg whites and antibiotics deplete biotin – though I doubt the Lipizzaners were indulging in too many of these, so it must be all that prancing around that puts a strain on their hooves.

White Spots They are quite common and often don't mean anything is wrong. They could be caused by a knock or can indicate lack of zinc or calcium.

Discoloured Nails Thickened yellow or even black nails are a sign you may have a fungal infection, although this tends to be more common in the toes. Fungal infections are the cause of most nail disorders and they can also be an indication that you have candida – an overgrowth of yeast in the body. Cut down on alcohol, sugars and acidic foods and take probiotics. Tea tree oil is a natural antiseptic; add five drops to a bowl of warm water and soak nails for about ten minutes daily. Discoloured nails can also be due to diabetes, prolonged illness or food intolerance, or even excess nicotine and nail varnish.

Pale Nails You could be suffering from anaemia – lack of iron – so eat more iron-rich foods, green leafy vegetables with vitamin C and meat, poultry and fish. Cut back on tea, coffee and wheat bran which can inhibit iron absorption. Pale nails are common in asthmatics who have difficulty getting enough oxygen.

Recipes

Food can make a big difference to your skin, by supplying essential vitamins, and minerals. A fibre-rich diet can prevent your liver and kidneys becoming overworked and expelling excess toxins through your skin, dulling your complexion. Fruit and vegetables provide antioxidants to mop up the free radicals produced by modern living. You can also feed your skin from the outside as well as the inside with fresh strawberry toners and avocado moisturisers – a new bargain range of cosmetics you have at your fingertips! I have included the most easy-to-apply accessible natural cosmetic recipes. I remember one summer, when I was in my twenties, massaging the flat's communal olive oil on to my legs and arms every night before I went to bed. It did work – my skin was a lovely glossy texture – in fact it was even remarked upon, but it was like sleeping in salad dressing every night and the sheets were a write-off, so it wasn't really worth it in the long term.

Antioxidant foods

Your skin is your biggest organ, so think how much oxidation is going on all the time. Mop up free radicals with plenty of antioxidant foods. Brightly coloured plants and vegetables are rich in antioxidants because the pigments which give them their colour are not purely aesthetic, they are to protect the plant from the sun's UV rays and other elements which could cause damage to the plant. By eating them we can also gain the same protection. It really is a case of thinking rainbow food: red, orange, yellow, green and purple. Try and have as colourful – literally – a diet as possible

- Red – tomatoes, red peppers, strawberries, cherries, grapes are rich in the antioxidant lycopene. Cooking actually makes it easier for your body to access lycopene so cooked tinned tomatoes have their benefits.
- Orange – oranges, mangoes, papayas, apricots, carrots, orange peppers and sweet potatoes are all rich in alpha and beta carotene which protects the skin from UV free radical damage.
- Yellow – sweetcorn, squash, yellow peppers, bananas and nectarines are rich in beta cryptothanxin which helps with the exchange of vitamins, minerals and fats between cells.
- Green – spinach, kale, broccoli, pears, apples, green grapes and green tea are all rich in lutein which is best known for its association with healthy eyes.
- Purple – aubergines, beetroot, plums, grapes and blueberries all contain anthocyanidins which have been found to prevent collagen from breaking down.

Orange Spectrum Seafood Chowder

Enjoy this thick stew of red and orange peppers and bright yellow sweetcorn. Not only are they gloriously colourful but the vegetables are also rich in lycopene, alpha carotene, beta carotene and beta cryptothanxin. There's protein, too, and some collagen-building lysine in the fish, especially the cod – so take that, wrinkles!

N.B. several reputable sources – e.g. Drs Murray and Pizzorno – state that lysine is required for collagen formation and repair of tissue as well as growth, hormones and enzymes, so all good for the skin.

Serves 4–6

Ingredients

125g butter
1 large Spanish onion, roughly chopped
1 red pepper, finely chopped
1 orange pepper, finely chopped
1 large leek, cut in 1cm slices on the diagonal
325g can sweetcorn, drained
1kg mix of mild-tasting fish (e.g. monkfish, halibut, turbot, cod, salmon) along with some small pieces of smoked salmon or smoked haddock and a few prawns

1 tablespoon vegetable oil
60g butter
40g plain or soya flour
900ml fish stock (including the juices from the cooked fish, above)
300ml double cream
sea salt and freshly ground black pepper
1 handful of parsley and tarragon, roughly chopped

Method

Melt 125g of butter and, over a low heat, gently fry the onion, peppers, leek and sweetcorn till just cooked (about 10 minutes). Set aside.

Chop the fish into rough chunks and cook gently in a large frying pan with the oil to prevent sticking; try not to break up the chunks of fish. When the fish is cooked but still moist and tender, strain off the pan juices and set aside. In a jug, add the pan juices to the fish stock to total 900ml.

Melt 60g of butter in a large, deep pot, sift over the flour and stir to a smooth paste/roux. Now add the hot fish stock and stir over a medium heat as the sauce thickens.

When the sauce base has thickened, stir in the fried vegetables then, gently, stir in the cooked fish. Pour in the cream, season with salt and pepper and warm through.

Immediately before serving, sprinkle over a handful of parsley mixed with tarragon. Don't let the chowder boil after the tarragon is added or it will lose its delicate flavour.

Looking Good Red Pepper and Parsley Green Pâté

Roasted, red, lycopene-rich peppers, parsley which is an excellent source of vitamin C and zinc-rich almonds are whizzed together with oil rich in essential fatty acids.

Use as a spread on toast or mix with a little yoghurt to make a dip.

Serves 4 as a starter

Ingredients

1 red pepper
75g flaked almonds
1 large bunch curly parsley, stalks removed

100g pitted green olives
juice of ½ lemon
75ml hemp or flaxseed oil

Method

Slice the red pepper in half longways and remove middle white part, cook under a hot grill with the skin side up, till soft but not blackened.

Toast the almonds in a dry frying pan till they colour – this happens very quickly so keep a watchful eye on them.

Put the peppers and almonds together with the remaining ingredients into a blender and whizz to a smoothish pâté.

Mediterranean Bake for a Beautiful Skin

Grated courgette gives a green vegetable crunch to the egg and cheese base which is rich in protein and vitamin D. Tomatoes and peppers with their antioxidant reds form the bright topping.

Delicious hot or cold – ideal for picnics and packed lunches.

Serves 3

Ingredients

Base

Olive oil and flour (for the baking tin)

2 courgettes

50g mozzarella

50g Parmesan cheese

2 eggs, beaten

50g wholemeal flour

fresh basil leaves

sea salt and freshly ground black pepper

Topping

4 tomatoes, sliced

2 red peppers, sliced

4 unpeeled garlic cloves, whole

olive oil to drizzle

Method

Preheat the oven to 180°C/350°F/Gas 4. Oil and lightly flour a 20cm square tin.

First, prepare the egg base. Grate the courgettes and cheese using a food processor or by hand, it doesn't matter if you get lumps of mozzarella, and put in a large mixing bowl. Add the eggs, sift in the flour, add some torn basil leaves, season with salt and pepper and mix to combine.

Put the mixture into the prepared tin, pat it down and set aside.

For the topping, in a shallow baking tray scatter the tomatoes, peppers and garlic cloves and drizzle with olive oil.

Put both the base and the topping in the oven and bake for 40 minutes – the topping should turn golden brown.

Spread the gooey red pepper and tomato topping over the base and serve hot or cold.

Purple Spectrum Beetroot Dip

Iron-rich beetroot is a great antioxidant. Serve this exotically spiced colourful dip with raw vegetable sticks or warm pitta bread for a full-on attack on cellular ageing.

Serves enough as a starter for 4

Ingredients

5 beetroot, boiled, skinned
   and roughly chopped
   (or buy vacuum-packed)
300ml plain yoghurt
2 garlic cloves, crushed
2 tablespoons lemon juice
2 tablespoons extra virgin olive oil

sea salt and freshly ground
   black pepper
½ teaspoon each of ground
   cumin, coriander, paprika
   and cinnamon

Method

Put all the ingredients in a blender and whizz to a smooth paste.

Forever Young Chicken, Beetroot and Orange Salad

Orange and purple antioxidants together with vitamin C in the vegetable and fruit, along with chunks of collagen-building protein and some good fats from oil and nuts, all add up to a very anti-ageing salad.

This recipe comes from the very youthful-looking Richard Barclay, managing director of the Rannoch Smokery in Perthshire where he produces the most wonderful smoked venison and chicken. Richard took me mountain biking and cooking in the Grampian mountains when we were filming *The Woman Who Ate Scotland*.

The smoked chicken – and the toasted cumin seeds – bring subtle earthiness to this dish but substitute cooked chicken breast if you can't source smoked chicken and the flavours still work.

Serves 4

Ingredients

Chicken, Beetroot and Orange Salad

250g boiled, skinned and sliced (or buy vacuum-packed) beetroot

2 oranges, peeled and chopped

handful of rocket

½ a cold-smoked chicken (or 2 cooked chicken breasts), cut in chunks

Dressing

2 teaspoons cumin seeds

2 teaspoons lemon juice

1 teaspoon honey

3 tablespoons olive oil

3 tablespoons pine nuts

Method

In a large serving bowl, combine the beetroot, oranges, rocket and chicken.

To make the dressing, first toast the cumin seeds in a dry frying pan until fragrant then pound in a pestle and mortar (or put in a small bowl and pound with the end of a rolling pin). Now, whisk together the lemon juice, honey and olive oil then mix in the pounded cumin and pour the spiced dressing over the salad.

Finally, toast the pine nuts in a dry frying pan and scatter over the salad.

Avocados are an excellent source of monosaturated fatty acids, potassium, vitamin B, E, glutathione and fibre. A ripe avocado should yield to soft pressure. Some supermarkets sell ready to eat avocados in plush protective packaging, but it is cheaper to buy them unripe and allow to ripen naturally at room temperature. To speed up the process, put the unripe avocados in a paper bag with a banana and the ethylene gas from the banana will ripen the avocado. Once ripe, you can keep avocados in the fridge. The avocado is a great friend of the skin, both eaten and applied externally, thanks to its rich oils, especially vitamin E which can slow down the ageing process. You can eat an avocado as a snack, neat with a little salt, pepper, omega 3, 6 or 9 oil and a touch of balsamic vinegar in the natural dip where the pit was. And keep the skin and use it as an on-the-spot moisturiser – see page 198.

Good-Looking Guacamole

I love this easy-to-make dip with corn chips, as a sandwich spread and in salads.

Makes for four as a dip

Ingredients

2 medium avocados
juice of half a lime
1 shallot, finely minced
2 garlic cloves, minced
½ teaspoon salt

1 small tomato, peeled (plunge in boiling water for 1 minute, then plunge briefly in cold water then peel), deseeded and finely chopped
few sprigs of fresh coriander, roughly roughly chopped

Method

Peel, slice and chop the avocado flesh and put it in a mixing bowl with lime juice, shallot, garlic, salt, tomato and coriander. Mix and crush with a fork so that some of the avocado breaks down but you still have a few small chunks.

Cover the bowl and keep in the fridge till ready to eat. You can also submerge the pit of the avocado in the guacamole as for some reason this is supposed to prevent the vibrant green avocado from darkening.

Smoked Mackerel Teriyaki Salad

A speedy-to-make dish which is rich in essential fatty acids and protein thanks to the mackerel and pumpkin seeds and lots of green leaves which support the liver. Here, the sauce for the fish doubles as a warm dressing for the salad leaves.

Beware of eating too many smoked products as they tend to have a high salt content – the recommended amount of salt is 6g per day for an adult.

Serves 2

Ingredients

2 tablespoons soy sauce

1 tablespoon rice wine or dry sherry

1 teaspoon maple syrup

1 clove garlic, chopped

½ onion, chopped

200g smoked mackerel fillet, flaked

50g rocket

1 handful pumpkin seeds

Method

In a small pan, mix all the ingredients up to and including the onion and heat till the sauce bubbles.

Cook, bubbling, for 1 minute then add the fish. Turn off heat and allow to stand in the pan for five minutes; the sauce will turn to a rich, dark brown.

Divide the rocket over two plates and scatter over pumpkin seeds. Spoon the fish, along with the sauce, over the leaves.

Egyptian Beanfeast

I first tasted a variation of this dish in Egypt where it is called *ful medames*, served for breakfast.

Review your breakfast options, break away from your usual cereal and start the day with this spicy, fibre-packed, toxin-removing beanfeast complete with slow-burn carbs and lycopene-rich tomatoes.

Incredibly quick to prepare, this recipe also works well as a lunch or supper dish served with brown rice or quinoa and steamed vegetables.

Serves 2–3

Ingredients

1 tablespoon olive oil
1 medium onion, chopped
1 teaspoon whole cumin seeds
1 teaspoon ground coriander
2 cloves garlic, crushed

400g can chopped or plum tomatoes
400g can mixed beans, drained
1 lime, quartered

Method

Heat the oil in a saucepan, cook the onion till soft then add the spices and garlic and cook for about 10 minutes. Add the tomatoes and beans and simmer for 20 minutes. Squeeze in the juice from one of the lime quarters; serve in bowls with the remaining lime quarters on the side.

Sulphur is an essential skin mineral as it is a constituent of keratin and collagen and keeps bonds between cells pliable. Sulphur is also needed for new cell formation since you make a new skin every twenty-eight days. Sulphur-rich foods include garlic, onions, eggs, legumes, Brussels sprouts, broccoli and cabbage, i.e. ones that have a tendency to make their presence known . . .

Hong Kong Broccoli Stir-Fry

I fell in love with this garlicky, crunchy broccoli dish in Hong Kong. Stir-frying is the best way to cook broccoli so that it keeps its crunch and high vitamin content.

My Cantonese vocabulary has shrunk so much since I don't use it anymore, but in a garlicky, Proustian moment the Cantonese for broccoli came back immediately to me: *sai lam fa*, which translates as 'western flower vegetable'.

Serve this fast-fried broccoli as a side dish or, for an all-in-one vegetable stir-fry meal, bump up the interest and sustenance factor by adding finely sliced carrots, green beans and celery.

Serves 2 as side dish

Ingredients

500g broccoli
2 tablespoons vegetable oil
2 garlic cloves, finely minced

1 knob ginger, peeled and
finely chopped
sea salt

Method

Break or cut off the broccoli florets from the stems and cut them into either halves or quarters. Discard any leaves and slice the stems thinly, 1cm thick across the diagonal. Plunge the prepared broccoli into a large pan of boiling water for 1 minute then drain completely.

Heat a wok or frying pan and add the oil. When the oil is smoking hot add the garlic and ginger. Then add the drained broccoli and stir-fry for 1–2 minutes so the broccoli is still crunchy. Sprinkle with salt to taste.

Ricotta Cake with Fruit

I love cooking with ricotta – it is made from whey, a by-product of butter-making, so it's relatively low fat. This creamy, lemon rind-flecked cake is low in fat as well as in sugar and flour.

The cake marries perfectly with antioxidant-rich fruits such as dark purple blueberries, ruby red raspberries, brilliant red strawberries or golden peaches. To cut down on sugar, I use rosewater to sweeten fruit but be light-handed, rosewater is quite strong!

Ricotta cake is an ideal pudding if you have eaten a relatively light veggie carbohydrate main course and so need to bump up the protein content of your meal.

Serves 4–6

Ingredients

250g ricotta
1 egg
50g sugar

½ tablespoon almond extract
pinch of salt
1 lemon: rind, finely grated;

25g plain flour   juice of ½ lemon

½ tablespoon vanilla extract

Method

Preheat the oven to 180°C/350°F/Gas 4. Grease and line the base and sides of a 20cm springform cake tin with baking paper.

Put all ingredients into a food processor and whizz till smooth and creamy (or put in a large mixing bowl and beat by hand).

Spoon the mixture into the prepared cake tin and bake in the centre of the oven for 30 minutes. The cake should be just leaving the edges of the tin and feel slightly firm to touch.

Leave the cake in the tin to cool then transfer to a plate and slice. Serve with any chopped fruits of your choice.

Glowing Skin Fruit Compote

This thick spicy compote is a great source of antioxidants. And don't peel the apples for this recipe, you'll lose the valuable fibre in the pectin.

Serve for breakfast with porridge, muesli or yoghurt, or try it with *Ricotta Cake*, see opposite.

Serves 4 as an accompaniment

Ingredients

1 large unpeeled cooking
   apple, Cox's or Granny
   Smiths
1 eating apple such as
   Cox's Orange Pippin
6 cardamom pods

1 stick cinnamon
3 slices ginger root
75ml cold water
100g fresh or frozen soft fruit
   e.g. raspberries, strawberries,
   blueberries (hulled)

Method

Core and cube the apples and put in a medium-sized pan. Snip the cardamom pods over the apples to extract the small dark seeds and discard the pods. Add the rest of the spices and water and simmer for 10 minutes, till the cooking apple has gone fluffy, but the eating one still has some shape. Hunt out the cinnamon stick and ginger slices. Add the fruit which turns the apple stew a gorgeous dark purple and serve either hot or cold.

Apricot and Almond Dessert

Fibre-rich apricots and almonds are also packed full of antioxidant beta carotene and healing zinc, so they're great for your skin.

When you're buying dried apricots, try to buy the dark-coloured, dried unsulphured apricots – as the fat orange ones may have been dried using sulphur dioxide which can cause stomach upsets.

Serves 2

Ingredients

150g dried, unsulphured
  apricots
2 tablespoons flaked almonds

150g thick, set Greek yoghurt
pinch of ground cinnamon

Method

In a bowl, pour warm water over the apricots to cover and soak overnight.

After soaking, stone the apricots. In a dry frying pan, toast the almonds till golden brown then crush lightly.

Divide the soaked apricots between 2 large wine glasses, spoon ½ the yoghurt into each glass then sprinkle with cinnamon and almonds. Chill for at least at hour before serving.

External Skin Treatments That Are Good Enough To Eat

Avocado skin treat

The oil hidden away in the peel of the avocado is a wonderful facial moisturiser. Lightly massage your face with the inside of the peel, using gentle upward strokes. Let the oil residue remain on your skin for about fifteen minutes, then wash your face gently with three or four rinses of tepid water and pat dry.

Avocado Dry Skin Food Fest

This is a lovely treat for dry skin and you should feel an immediate improvement in texture.

Ingredients

1 egg yolk   ½ avocado

Method

Whisk the egg yolk till it is light and frothy then add the avocado to form a smooth cream (you could mix with a hand blender).

Cleanse your skin using your usual cleansing methods, then smooth the avocado cream evenly all over your face and neck.

Relax with the cream on for about 20 minutes. Wipe off with a face cloth soaked in clear, tepid water followed by a quick rinse of cold water.

Avocado Oily Skin Tonic

This is great for oily skin: the oatmeal exfoliates while the egg white helps to dry up excess oil.

Ingredients

½ avocado

1 egg white

1 heaped tablespoon fine oatmeal

Method

Mash the avocado to a pulp and blend together with the egg white and oatmeal (you could mix with a hand blender).

Cleanse your skin using your usual cleansing methods, before smoothing the avocado cream evenly all over your face.

Relax with the cream on for about 20 minutes. Rinse off with warm water.

Oatmeal Skin Polish

'Polishing' or stimulating skin helps to clean pores and it can also improve peripheral circulation and, therefore, oxygen delivery; it may also improve lymphatic drainage. Beware, however, of over-harsh exfoliation and scrubs which can irritate your skin.

This recipe makes a gentle exfoliant to use on your face and neck – add some pinhead oatmeal if you want a rougher texture to use on legs or arms.

For an oatmeal hand wash, add water instead of oil to the oatmeal; just keep a small jar of coarse oatmeal near the sink.

Ingredients

2 teaspoons fine oatmeal   1 teaspoon almond oil

Method

Mix the oatmeal and oil to a smooth paste, splash some warm water on your face and neck and apply the paste moving upwards, then remove with warm water and pat dry with a towel.

Ginger Cellulite Scrub

This is a delicious-smelling body scrub intended to stimulate peripheral blood circulation.

Ingredients

2 teaspoons ginger, grated   few drops of almond oil
2 tablespoons sea salt   (optional)

Method

Mix together the ginger and salt then massage into areas of skin affected by cellulite. If necessary, to ease the massage add a few drops of almond oil.

Strawberry Face Pack

Give your skin a boost with this simple, easy-to-use, summer skin lift. Strawberries contain vitamins B, C, E and K.

Apply two fresh, crushed strawberries to your face and leave for 15 minutes, splash with water to remove.

External hair treatments

The oils that feed your skin will also feed your hair, so moisturise your hair with warm olive oil before shampooing and gently massage your scalp with almond or coconut oil to stimulate the circulation to the follicles. To add a gloss, steep the juice of half a lemon in a cup of boiling water and rinse hair in the lemon-scented liquid after shampooing; there is no need to rinse again in water. This is how a conditioner works, as it restores the acid/alkali balance to the hair, making it look more shiny.

Hot Ginger Oil Treatment

This is great for damaged hair and can also help prevent dandruff.

Ingredients

3 tablespoons olive oil

2 teaspoons ginger, grated

Method

Heat the oil and ginger in a pan till it reaches blood temperature – this helps it penetrate the hair shaft better (or, if you don't like the 'ginger bits', infuse and strain then heat to blood temperature).

Massage through your hair and into your scalp then wrap your hair in a warm towel for about 10 minutes. Shampoo and rinse thoroughly.

Peppermint Footbath

This is an invigorating bath to stimulate blood flow to the feet and the almond oil will also moisturise.

Ingredients

1 teaspoon almond oil
3 drops peppermint essential
oil

warm water

Method

Add the oils to a feet-sized bowl of warm water and soak your feet for 5 minutes. To further stimulate circulation, put some smooth pebbles in the base of the bowl and roll your feet over them.

Ginger Footbath

Ginger is thought to be a great circulation booster. This footbath requires very little effort to prepare and it's ideal when you are cold and want to promote an all-over warm, inner glow.

Ingredients

2 teaspoons ground ginger and   warm water
  2cm chopped root ginger

Method

Add the gingers to a feet-sized bowl of warm water and soak your feet till the water cools.

Good Skin Checklist

- Cut back on sugar, alcohol, caffeine, saturated fats.
- Eat plenty of brightly coloured fruit and vegetables.
- Increase zinc-rich foods – oysters, almonds, fish and eggs.
- Drink water, about one and a half litres per day.
- Enjoy unsaturated fats found in seeds and nuts which are also a good source of zinc and protein, and oily fish. Use

omega oil in smoothies or salad dressing or take as a supplement.

- Vitamin E, also known as alpha-tocopherol, is found in almonds, in many oils including wheat germ, safflower, corn and soybean oils, and also in mangoes, nuts, broccoli and other foods, so don't miss out.
- Make sure you have a little protein at every meal for good keratin formation.
- Protect your skin against the sun.
- Do at least thirty minutes exercise to get your heart delivering oxygen to your skin cells and even a bit of a sweat will trigger the production of sebum which acts as your skin's own moisturiser. Exercise also helps manage insulin and blood sugar levels which are both damaging to the collagen in the dermis.

Have a Good Skin Day!

Breakfast: eat like an Egyptian and start the day with cumin-spicy beans – a good source of soluble fibre which will help expel toxins.

Snack: avocado dip with carrot sticks, you get vitamin E from the avocado and vitamin C from the carrot sticks.

Lunch: mackerel teriyaki salad which is a source of good fats, protein and greens.

Snack: apple – lots of pectin, fibre and vitamin C.

Supper: Mediterranean bake with toxin-removing fibre and protein-rich egg. Serve with a green salad tossed in pumpkin oil and pumpkin seeds. Ricotta cake with strawberries and raspberries – protein-charged cake with fruit.

Make a face pack from two crushed strawberries left over from pudding and you could also use the avocado skin for a mid-morning moisturise (see foodie external treatments, page 198).

Drink at least one and a half litres of water, neat or as herbal teas – nettle is great for circulation.

Take a brisk walk outside – so your cheeks are a healthy pink.

Bonuses: all that filling fibre and vegetables plus less junk food could mean that, if you are overweight, you lose some weight. Your immune system will be stronger and you may be less likely to catch colds, apart from being in a better position to fight off more serious attacks on your body's cells. Vitamin E is great for heart health and circulation – so blood pressure could go down – and there is less chance of getting varicose veins, the last thing you want when you have lovely smooth slim legs. And exercise is a great de-stresser, so you will be in a happy frame of mind.

Foods That Hurt – and Those That Heal

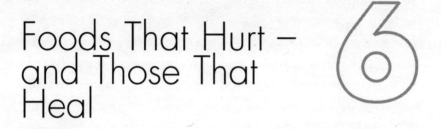

It was one of those great-to-be-alive winter mornings; sunglasses-on-dazzling-blue sky, thick-pile carpets of freshly fallen snow and not a Gore-Texed skier in sight. I was blissfully skiing down a mountain in the French Alps at full speed, without a care in the world. Then I suddenly realised I was going too fast and the piste was getting steeper and steeper; I tried to stop, hit thick powder, missed a tree and heard a wrenching sound as I tore the cruciate ligament in my left knee. Unable to move or ski, I was blood-wagoned off the mountain to a French doctor who pronounced my condition *'terminée'* – my skiing, not my leg. I spent Christmas Eve with my leg in plaster in my bedroom above the bar where I worked, while everyone else was downstairs getting 'plastered' in the more conventional sense.

As a result of my skiing accident, I lost my job and, determined not to return home so early on in my 'snow bunny' career, hopped off round the village looking for alternative employment until my leg healed. Luckily for me, some chalet owners had been let down by their chalet girl and I persuaded them that I could be a very able one-legged replacement. And so I found myself thrust into the heat of the kitchen with fifteen hungry skiers to feed three times a day: breakfast, afternoon tea and a three-course evening meal – and only one leg to stand on. I asked the other chalet girls for recipes that had survived a thorough testing under the most rigorous conditions on ravenous skiers, using as few francs as possible, three thousand feet above sea level with a temperamental oven not to mention a temperamental cook. When I came back from France I tried to interest publishers in a book called *Cooking For Fifteen On One Leg* as I had so many handy, easy recipes. They all said 'no', with one saying they thought I was aiming at a very limited market . . .

At the time, I had no idea what to eat to heal my torn ligament. More concerned with feeding hungry skiers, I ploughed into cooking and inevitably found myself eating French mountain food – copious bottles of red wine, bread, mountain cheese, cream, pasta, cakes and biscuits – all the while hopping about with one leg in plaster. A month later, my plaster was off, and after a bit of physiotherapy, I was able to ski again and thought no more of the accident.

Yet, over the years I noticed that occasionally after a night out involving alcohol and rich food, my left knee would become very stiff and inflamed, yet I couldn't understand why. I blamed my late night or uncoordinated dancing on my inability to walk the next day. It wasn't until I started to study nutrition that I realised the incredible effect perfectly innocent-sounding food can have on the body in terms of helping it heal or causing it harm.

'Itis'

After a particularly bad flare-up of my left knee, I limped along to a doctor who said I had developed arthritis in my knee and, short of getting a knee replacement, all I could do was to take anti-inflammatories when it got too bad. At thirty-one I was appalled to think I had arthritis but, as I learned, arthritis is no respecter of age. Arthritis is a term broadly used to cover more than two hundred different illnesses – all involving degeneration of the joints and soft tissues – and it can strike at any age. 'Itis' means inflammation and 'arthro' means joints, so basically I was suffering from inflamed joints. My arthritis was caused by injury to the cruciate knee ligaments which are a strong band of fibrous tissues which bind the femur and tibia bones together at the knee. I can't heal the damage – the ligament will never knit back together completely – and the soft tissues round my knee are damaged. And it is sadly a documented fact that cruciate injury may trigger osteo-arthritis in later life. Osteoarthritis is most common in older people, caused by inevitable long-term wear and tear of the joints, so most people over sixty have some symptoms of arthritis. Unlike so many of our diseases, it is of little comfort to know it is not a modern disease; archaeologists have found dinosaur and Neanderthal skeletons with evidence of arthritic bones.

This Could Help Your 'Itis'

If your biggest burst of exercise is hunting for the remote control, don't abandon me now, this chapter isn't just about eating for arthritis sufferers; it is all about eating foods that don't aggravate any type of inflammation in your body. This covers so many conditions from

If your biggest burst of exercise is hunting for the remote control, don't abandon me now

sunburn, which is a type of inflammation when your skin goes red in reaction to the ultraviolet rays of sunshine, to other skin inflammations such as psoriasis, eczema and acne. Inflammation also covers internal complaints such as bronchitis – which is inflammation of the bronchial tubes – period pain, endometriosis, phlebitis and cystitis; even a sprained wrist. Anything with an 'itis' refers to any inflammation in your body. Some allergies express themselves as inflammation caused by what should be a harmless or at least non-infectious agent. So adopting an anti-inflammatory diet may help in some cases.

Some foods can actually cause inflammation – junk foods, high-fat meats, sugar and fast foods will all increase inflammation in the body. This is partially due to the unhealthy fats used in preparing and processing these foods, especially trans fats and saturated fats. Saturated fats are also found in meats, dairy products and eggs. While all of these foods are important sources of minerals and vitamins, you don't need the extra saturated fat. These foods also contain fatty acids called arachidonic acid. While some arachidonic acid is essential for your health, too much of it may make any potential inflammation worse by causing irritation to vulnerable areas. High-fat foods and other acid-causing foods make the body acidic which also contributes to inflammation.

Prostaglandins

Essential Fatty Acids (EFAs) in food – oils, nuts, meat, fish and dairy – are broken down into prostaglandins. Prostaglandins are key to the whole inflammatory process. Prostaglandins are short-lived substances that act like hormones. They behave like regulators and chemical messengers and are produced locally by the cells when they are needed and afterwards are quickly broken down. They affect the tissue immediately round them either in a good or bad way.

There are three families or series of prostaglandins: series one and three are anti-inflammatory, and also help reduce cholesterol, lower blood pressure, relax blood vessels, decrease inflammation and pain, improve nerve function and help insulin work. Series two prostaglandins, however, promote inflammation in the body and are derived from arachidonic acid. Arachidonic acid is also found in meat and dairy, which is why excess red meat and dairy can cause inflammation. The key to inflammation is to try to reduce prostaglandins series two and encourage series one and three. And how do you do that? By increasing essential fatty acids in your diet.

Essential Fatty Acids

EFAs are so called because they are essential to your body and your body can't make them. EFAs are also referred to as omega fatty acids. Omega means 'great' in Greek as they do so much – and they really do. EFAs are converted to prostaglandins series one and three, which can lower blood pressure, decrease inflammation, improve function of your nervous and immune systems, help insulin work, support your vision, coordination, support your skin cell membranes and nourish your brain. The science behind EFAs does seem to make sense and they are an easy economical addition to your diet.

Fats

Firstly your body needs fat; fat is good, fats help you to absorb fat-soluble vitamins, make energy, they act as insulation, control passage of compounds in and out of cells, ensure healthy nerve tissue and form powerful hormones. All fats or lipids contain various combinations of carbon, hydrogen and oxygen. Some fats are saturated. This means there are single bonds between all the carbon atoms and they are not easily broken – they tend to be solid like butter. Monounsaturated means there is only one double carbon bond, olive oil for example. Saturated and monounsaturated fats are not essential nutrients, whereas polyunsaturated fats such as omegas, which have more than one double bond, are essential to your body.

Most foods that contain fat have a mixture of all three; meat is mainly saturated fat but it does have some mono- and polyunsaturated fats. Omega oils are polyunsaturated as they all have one or more double carbon bond. The number which comes after the omega such as 3, 6, or 9 merely indicates where the first double carbon bond is – whether it's on the third carbon atom or the sixth or ninth. Your body processes the omega fatty acids in different ways or pathways depending on where the bond is. It is the breakdown of the EFAs which is important to your body.

Omega 6

Omega 6 is found in sunflower seeds, sesame seeds, pumpkin seeds, almonds, pecans, soya bean and walnuts. With some help from certain vitamins and enzymes, it gets broken down to gamma-linolenic acid (GLA), and ultimately prostaglandin series one. Series one prostaglandin helps prevent blockage and clots in the blood. By keeping the blood thin it relaxes blood vessels and helps maintain water balance in your body. GLA is also very useful for inflamed skin conditions – but can aggravate epilepsy.

PMT

Gamma-linolenic acid (GLA) has wonderful hormone balance qualities and can make a real difference in easing pre-menstrual breast pain. GLA is also very useful at preventing an increase in series two prostaglandins which are a cause of period pain. GLA is best consumed through borage and evening primrose oil supplements as less GLA gets processed from the seeds and oils. In addition evening primrose oil is rich in botanical triterpenes which are hormone-like substances which may boost the immune system and could help if you are feeling rundown during menstruation.

Omega 3

Omega 3s are predominantly found in oily fish such as salmon, mackerel, tuna and herring, and pumpkin seeds, linseeds or flaxseeds. Once you have chomped on your salad dressed with flaxseed oil your body, with some help from enzymes and vitamins, breaks down the omega 3 which is then converted into an acid called eicosapentaenoic acid EPA (found in fish) then to docosahexaenoic acid DHA (also found in fish) which is finally converted to a prostaglandin series three. Prostaglandin series three are essential for brain function as well as to boost the immune system, metabolism and reduce inflammation. Hemp oil is a very rich source of vegetarian omega 3 fatty acids and also contains substantial amounts of omega 6 fatty acids. Hemp contains a good balance of omega 3 and omega 6.

Most of us can make prostaglandins from both omega 3 and 6 fatty acids but if you have a family history of allergies you may be unable to convert them. In which case you should buy the already converted GLA and EPA supplements. Like all things in your body, nothing works alone and you also need vitamin B6, magnesium, biotin, calcium and zinc to make conversions, so you still need a healthy balanced diet which includes wholegrains and green leafy vegetables.

How Much Fat?

Your ideal diet should not consist of more than thirty per cent fat, the majority of which should be unsaturated (your brain is composed of sixty per cent fat and cell membranes need fat to keep their shape). Saturated fats should account for no more than ten per cent of your diet. You definitely need omega 3 and omega 6 fatty acids and there is discussion about the ratio, but most experts have settled on a ratio of one part omega 3 to three parts omega 6. But it is quite easy to get enough balanced omegas; you only need to eat about one or two tablespoons of flaxseed oil per day – add to smoothies, cereal, salad dressing or even take on a spoon like cod liver oil medicine. By the way, cod liver oil may contain high amounts of vitamin A but you have to be sure that it is free of mercury. Fish oil capsules are a safer bet. Or take two or three tablespoons of ground seeds; they need to be ground otherwise the seed's intact protective outer layer can pass unscathed through your digestion process and you won't get any benefit. Grind two parts linseed (also called flaxseed) with one part sesame, pumpkin and pumpkin seeds in a coffee grinder and add to cereals and smoothies. Also eat two 125g portions of oily fish every week.

Trans Fats

There has been much debate about trans fats and how to avoid them. Why? Well, they are artificially created through a process called hydrogenation which means your body cannot process them. Manufacturers like using trans fats as they are more solid and stable than oils and are less likely to spoil, so give food a longer shelf life. They also have a less greasy feel.

Many food manufacturers have stopped using trans fats due to health concerns about their possible link to raised cholesterol, but you will still find them in processed foods such as biscuits, cakes and fried foods. Look out for the words 'partially hydrogenated' or shortening. Trans fat may increase inflammation in the body through the formation of fatty blockages in heart blood vessels and by preventing omega 3s doing their work. They also appear to damage the cells lining blood vessels, leading to inflammation. The simple way to avoid them is not to eat processed food and deep fried foods, and don't use partially hydrogenated oils or shortening when cooking.

Butter Butter is high in saturated fat (no double bonds between the carbon atoms) and cholesterol, but your body needs some saturated fat – no more than ten per cent per day – so don't feel guilty if you have a little bit of butter on your rye toast!

Fully Hydrogenated Vegetable Oil

Exposing liquid oils rich in unsaturated fats to hydrogen gas for a longer time makes hard, waxy, fully hydrogenated fats. They become saturated fats, and are completely trans fat-free, but they are still classed as saturated fats.

Traditional Liquid Vegetable Oils

No

The healthiest cooking oils are liquid vegetable oils such as olive, corn, rapeseed or sunflower oils. Remember, you can't cook with omega 3 and omega 6 oils as they tend to form damaging free radicals when heated, so use these traditional vegetable oils for stir frying. *Avocado. or ghee / Coconut oil are much better.*

Other Inflammatory Foods

On a recce for filming *The Woman Who Ate Scotland*, we spent a few days eating rabbit, hare and venison in Perthshire in autumn – which was heaven – until the next day when my knee had become very inflamed. I couldn't walk and could hardly bend it to get in the car, let alone get on a bike. I learned that game for me is inflammatory. A substance in game called purine increases the level of uric acid in my joints which irritates my already sensitive knee. Purines are also found in herring and shellfish, so it is a case of experimenting with foods and recording any ill effects to establish if you are sensitive to them. Processed meats such as luncheon meats, hot dogs and sausages contain chemicals called nitrites that can also cause increased inflammation.

For many people it is a case of trial and error. Some nutritionists would advise avoiding all gluten-containing products, because gluten is one of the most common causes of food allergies and sensitivities. Gluten is a protein in plants that the human body does not use. Gluten will damage nutrient-absorbing villi in the gut so that fewer nutrients can be absorbed. Sensitivities to gluten can include migraine and joint swelling. For me to rule out all gluten would rule out rye, barley and oats which I love, and luckily I don't get a reaction (bloating, sore stomach, inflamed joints etc.) to the proteins in rye and oats, but I do try to avoid wheat as the protein in wheat may aggravate my knee; furthermore its over-processed features can aggravate the gut.

Nightshade vegetables – potatoes, aubergines, tomatoes and peppers – can also aggravate joint swelling. The substance solanine found in them can cause pain in the joints of susceptible people, although I haven't found this. Again it is up to you to experiment and keep a food diary if you suffer from any kind of inflammation. Arthritis sufferers are also advised to steer clear of citrus fruits as they are acid forming, but again it is up to you to try out, as they are also a valuable source of vitamin C which is itself an anti-inflammatory.

For most people, dairy, wheat and saturated fats are acid forming and cause inflammation as opposed to wholefoods such as most fruit, vegetables and pulses which are alkaline forming. In general, it is good to avoid too much acid-forming food. I have noticed that excess wheat, dairy, red meat and game aggravate the pain in my knee most. However, what I have found – which is far more exciting – is that certain foods can make the condition better, to the point that – touch (sustainable) wood – I am not even aware of any pain in my knee and can still ski, play tennis and hike with no ill effects.

Now for the Good News

As well as omega 6- and omega 3-rich foods, such as oily fish, nuts and seeds, most fruits – all green vegetables, onions, garlic, spices especially turmeric, cardamom, cinnamon, ginger, coriander and cumin – have an anti-inflammatory effect. Most pulses and gluten-free grains such as brown rice, quinoa and buckwheat also have anti-inflammatory properties, so there are plenty of foods to choose from for an anti-inflammatory diet. These foods are also good sources of vitamins, minerals, protein, carbohydrate, fat and fibre, which your body needs for all its other processes.

Anti-inflammatory foods

These foods will help to reduce inflammation in your body as well as promote tissue healing and reduce tissue damage and pain. Even if you don't suffer from any obvious inflammation, they are all good food-habit suggestions.

- Papaya, cherries, blueberries, strawberries and other red-blue berries. In season, try and eat ten fresh cherries daily to help reduce pain and inflammation.
- Celery and celery seeds help prevent flare-ups.
- Ginger and turmeric inhibit pain-producing prostaglandins.
- Eat plenty of green leafy vegetables, and vegetables of every colour, plus non-citrus fresh fruit.
- Eat foods rich in calcium – be wary of dairy, so fill up on sesame seeds, dried figs and broccoli and leafy greens.
- Eat wholegrains (except wheat) such as spelt, kamut, millet and brown rice. Experiment with new grains.
- Eat oily fish, such as mackerel, herring, salmon and sardines.
- Eat fresh (not dried or tinned) pineapple as the enzyme bromelain found in the core of the pineapple will help reduce inflammation.
- Get your iron from food, but if you are taking multi-mineral supplements check to see if they contain extra iron (unless

your doctor tells you you're anaemic) as there is some evidence iron may be involved in pain, swelling and joint destruction.

- Bio flavanoids support vitamin C production which is anti-inflammatory, so include squash, broccoli, kale and dark berries which help with the production of good prosta-glandins.
- Avocados, sesame seeds, pumpkin seeds and sunflower seeds are all rich in vitamin E which can calm inflammation.

Cut back, or be wary of:

- Citrus fruits, wheat and shellfish. These can all trigger allergy-related inflammation. As can dairy products (experiment with different kinds of non-dairy milk such as oat, soy and almond milk).
- Be wary of the nightshade family: potatoes, tomatoes, peppers, aubergines, courgettes. Try eating them as a meal and look for any inflammatory signs; if not, then you are not affected by solanine. It would be a shame to ban them from your diet, as they are such a good source of vitamin C and antioxidants.
- Excess salt.
- Trans fats, saturated fats as well as sugar, stress and alcohol and low protein diets can all inhibit the enzymes that convert omega 3 fatty acid to DHA and EPA.

Recipes

The recipes and advice can benefit everyone. If you suffer from any kind of inflammation in your body – arthritis, hay fever, food allergies – or have suffered an accident, anything from breaking a bone to pulling a muscle, period pain, even having overdone the sunbathing (which is a kind of inflammation), try avoiding some of the most obvious inflammation-aggravating foods. Try cooking and eating delicious foods that heal.

Omega oils

Supermarkets and health food shops stock a good variety of omega oils. Experiment with flavours – flaxseed oil and hemp oil (great sources of omega 3, 6 and 9) both have distinct nutty tastes. Pumpkin seed oil is a gloriously dark green and is rich like its seeds. It is fun to match the seed to its oil when making a green salad. Sprinkle it with pumpkin seeds and dress with pumpkin seed oil and a pinch of lemon juice or toasted walnuts with leaves and walnut oil. The omega oils are unstable oils, so store them away from sunlight. They are best kept in the fridge and don't use them for cooking, as the heat will convert them to evil arachidonic acid, but they are great for salad dressing, whizzed into dips and drizzled on garlicky toast.

Breakfast: a cunning way to increase omega 3 and 6 for you and your family is to add ground seeds to breakfast cereal or smoothies. I like to soak linseeds for five minutes in warm water until they swell up, or crack them in a pestle and mortar and add them to porridge or muesli – they are also a great source of fibre.

Olé Tomatoes on Toast

Do as the Spanish do and rub toasted bread with a cut clove of raw garlic, squashed tomatoes and drizzle with oil. This versatile snack called *pan con tomate* can take you from breakfast, lunch, to pre-dinner canapé or a light, tasty supper.

Serves 1 as a snack

Ingredients

1 large tomato, cut in half
2 slices wholemeal or rye
   bread, toasted (slightly stale
   bread works best)

1 garlic clove cut in half
hemp oil or olive oil

Method

Rub the cut clove of garlic all over the hot toast then squish the tomato flesh down hard on to the garlic toast so the juice, seeds and flesh run over the toast, and drizzle with your chosen oil.

Pasta with Broccoli and Anchovies

Broccoli is an excellent source of calcium as well as vitamins K and C and it also contains some omega 3 essential fatty acids. The darker the floret, the more vitamins it contains. Anchovies contain omega 3-rich oil.

Serves 4

Ingredients

450g non-wheat pasta	6 garlic cloves, thinly sliced
450g broccoli, cut in bite-sized florets	4–6 anchovy fillets, drained and finely chopped
3 tablespoons olive oil	Parmesan cheese, freshly grated

Method

Cook the pasta according to pack instructions till *al dente*.

Meanwhile drop the broccoli into a pan of fast-boiling water and blanch for 1 minute. Drain and plunge into very cold water to stop it cooking further.

Heat the olive oil in a large frying pan, add the garlic and sauté till golden brown. Add the broccoli and anchovies and sauté for a couple of minutes more.

Drain the cooked pasta, return it back to its pot, add the broccoli and anchovy mix. Serve with freshly grated Parmesan.

Chalet Girl Turkey in Peanut Sauce

Ironically, the food I had easiest access to when I was in the French Alps – cheese, meat, dairy – was packed full of arachidonic acid (too much can cause inflammation). We were hundreds of miles from the sea so there was no oily fish. It was winter so there were few fresh vegetables and the French have not really embraced brown rice or brown bread.

I was given a version of this recipe by a chalet girl named Beci but, here, is an 'anti-inflammatory' adaptation of Beci's original.

Peanut butter was not easy to find in the local *supermarché* so we had to make our own; instead of adding olive oil to the nuts I've gone for flaxseed oil – a major source of omega 3s which are so important in calming the inflammatory pathways. Instead of cow's milk, I substituted non-dairy milks such as quinoa, rice and soy which work just as well. Turkey is a tasty yet low-fat, high-protein meat.

Serve with brown rice and green salad.

Serves 4

Ingredients

50g wholemeal or oat soya flour, seasoned

4 turkey or chicken escalopes

50g unsalted butter

300ml chicken stock

450ml semi skimmed cow's milk or soy or quinoa milk

100g salted roasted peanuts

3 tablespoons flaxseed oil

sea salt

Method

Put the seasoned flour in a plastic bag and toss the escalopes in it. Melt 25g butter in a frying pan and fry the floured escalopes till lightly browned. Remove the escalopes and keep warm while you make the sauce.

Melt the remaining butter then stir in the seasoned flour to make a thick paste. Gradually add the chicken stock and the milk till the sauce boils and thickens.

Make the peanut butter by whizzing together in a blender the peanuts, flaxseed oil and a pinch of sea salt.

Add the blended peanuts to the sauce. Serve the warm sauce over the turkey.

Joint-Friendly Veggie Moussaka

This is a fantastic mix of anti-inflammatory and healing spices: ginger, turmeric, cumin and cinnamon. Turmeric contains curcumin which gives the spice its brilliant yellow colour and also has anti-inflammatory properties. Ginger also contains very potent anti-inflammatory compounds called gingerols which inhibit formation of inflammatory cytokines – chemical messengers in the immune system. Cumin can stimulate the digestion, so is essential for encouraging proper digestion and assimilating nutrients. Cinnamon has a long history of being used as a medicine – some scientifically substantiated as being good for mediating blood sugar levels as well as helping circulation and digestion.

All the vegetables – courgettes, aubergines and mushrooms – help create an alkaline balance in the body; it is important to maintain a proper equilibrium between acid and alkali in the blood and body fluids. A slightly alkaline balance is preferred. Aubergines love to soak up oil but baking them avoids this and they develop an attractive, crisp quality.

Add a splash of colour by serving with a tomato salad dressed with a seed oil.

N.B. There are quite a few nightshade vegetables (see page 216) here, so don't make if you know that you react badly to the veg.

Serves 6

Ingredients

2 tablespoons ground cumin
2 tablespoons ground ginger
1 tablespoon turmeric

1 garlic clove, chopped
100ml red wine (optional)
2 x 400g cans plum tomatoes

2 tablespoons ground
   cinnamon
2 teaspoons freshly grated
   nutmeg
85g wholemeal or soya flour
100ml soya milk
2 aubergines, sliced
4 tablespoons olive oil
1 large onion, chopped

3 tablespoons tomato paste
1 handful of parsley, stalks
   removed and chopped
100g flaked almonds, toasted
100g dried, unsulphured
   apricots, chopped
100g raisins
450g courgettes, sliced
225g mushrooms, sliced

Yoghurt Topping

2 eggs, beaten
450ml natural yoghurt
2 tablespoons lemon juice
1 handful of fresh mint, chopped

75g Parmesan cheese,
   freshly grated

Method

Preheat the oven to 190°C/375°F/Gas 5.

On a flat plate, mix half of all the spices with the flour. Pour the milk into a shallow bowl and dip aubergine slices in milk, then the seasoned flour and arrange on an oiled baking sheet. Bake in the oven for 25 minutes till crisp.

Meanwhile, make the tomato sauce. Heat 3 table-spoons of the oil in a large frying pan, sauté the onion till soft, then add the garlic and gently fry. Add the wine and cook to reduce a little for about 5 minutes. Stir in the tomatoes, tomato paste and parsley and simmer for 30 minutes. Stir in the remainder of the spices plus the almonds and dried fruit and set aside.

In a separate frying pan, heat the remaining oil and fry the courgettes and mushrooms. Set aside.

Make the yoghurt topping: combine the eggs, yoghurt, lemon juice and mint.

Reduce the oven temperature to 170°C/325°F/Gas 3.

Now create your layered moussaka. Lay half the aubergines in a large, shallow ovenproof dish, follow this with a layer of fried courgettes and mushrooms, then a layer of tomato sauce. Add another layer of fried courgettes and mushrooms, another layer of tomato sauce and then finish with the remaining aubergines. Pour the yoghurt topping over the layered vegetables, sprinkle with Parmesan and bake for 45 minutes.

Pineapple

Fresh pineapple is a great source of bromelain which is a protein-digesting enzyme. It is an effective anti-inflammatory agent as it interacts with the prostaglandins which cause pain and it is thought that bromelain inhibits them and also seems to produce anti-inflammatory prostaglandins. Bromelain can also break down insoluble proteins such as fibrin which is associated with fluid retention. Bromelain is concentrated in the core of the pineapple, so cut a pineapple into 3cm slices, remove the skin from the edges and chop the whole slice and eat. Make pineapple rings a thing of the past.

Spiced-up Pineapple and Tofu Curry

Ginger, turmeric and pineapple contain the enzyme bromelain which is thought to be beneficial for some inflammatory conditions while tofu is a good, low-fat source of protein.

This curry is adapted from a recipe by Tom Kime, who uses lots of Asian spices. Don't be put off by the tofu, I've cooked this dish for confirmed carnivores who had to admit that they liked it.

Serve this pretty, green and golden curry with brown rice or quinoa.

Serves 2–3

Ingredients

Spice Paste

knob of ginger, peeled and grated
2 red chillies, deseeded
   and finely chopped
3 garlic cloves, chopped
1 small onion, chopped

Pineapple and Tofu Curry

2 tablespoons vegetable oil
1 teaspoon turmeric
500ml hot water
500g tofu, cut in chunks
juice of half a lime
½ teaspoon salt
1 teaspoon sugar

1 fresh pineapple, peeled,
   and cut in bite-sized pieces
250g green frozen or fresh
   beans
fresh coriander, stalks
   removed and chopped

Method

Make the spice paste in a blender. Add a splash of water and whizz all the ingredients to make a thickish paste.

To make the curry, heat 1 tablespoon of the oil in a large saucepan, fry the spice paste and add the turmeric. Then pour in the water and simmer for about 10 minutes.

Meanwhile, in a separate pan, heat the other tablespoon of oil and fry the tofu till golden brown.

Add the lime juice, salt, sugar and pineapple to the spice paste. Then add the beans (straight from the freezer if frozen) and fried tofu and simmer gently, taking care not to break up the tofu.

Serve sprinkled with chopped coriander.

No Pain Celery and Ginger Stir-Fry

Celery contains a compound called luteolin, an antioxidant thought to possess anti-inflammatory properties. Celery also contains vitamin C which may prevent free radical damage which, in turn, can trigger inflammation. Ginger may inhibit pain-producing prostaglandins.

Enjoy this stir-fry with brown rice or quinoa or serve with any meat or fish dish.

Serves 2–3

Ingredients

1–2 tablespoons vegetable oil
1 head celery, stalks cut into
   1cm diagonal slices
knob of fresh ginger, chopped
3 spring onions, thinly sliced
sea salt and freshly ground
   black pepper

2 tablespoons dry sherry
1 teaspoon soy sauce
1 teaspoon tomato paste
½ teaspoon unrefined
   golden caster sugar
1 teaspoon ground ginger
2 tablespoons flaked almonds

Method

Heat the oil in a large wok or frying pan, add the sliced celery, fresh ginger and spring onions then cook for about 10 minutes, until the celery is soft but still crunchy.

In a small bowl, mix together the salt, pepper, sherry, soy sauce, tomato paste, sugar and ground ginger then add to the fried celery and stir-fry for 2 minutes. Sprinkle in the flaked almonds, stir to mix through and serve.

Fish

Oily fish such as mackerel, herring, lake trout, salmon, tuna, sardines and anchovies all have high levels of omega 3s, but white fish such as cod also has some. You should try to eat two or three 125g portions of fish a week to get your recommended dose of EPA and DHA. A lot of people don't like fish because of its texture, bones and dull flavour, but do think again and try these delicious fish recipes, zapped up with spices and marinades. The joy of fish is that it cooks very quickly so it is great healthy 'fast food'. Overcooking is the worst crime you can commit against a fish. Most oily fish is sustainable and there have been attempts to farm cod on Shetland. Freezing does spoil the texture – bought frozen fish is better than home frozen; home freezing is too slow and can spoil the texture. Try and buy fresh and use on the day or buy frozen and keep frozen until ready to use.

Anchovy and Sesame-Topped Tuna

This is a very pretty and quick to make sophisticated dish – bright parsley green and anchovy breadcrumb topping on lightly grilled tuna steaks. Anchovies and fresh tuna are good sources of omega 3s. Be wary of eating tuna more than once a week, as too much can cause mercury to build up in your body. The Food Standards Agency advises: no more than four medium-sized cans or two fresh tuna steaks per week. Sesame seeds are a good omega 6 source.

Serve the fish with grilled red peppers (cook them, while you are cooking the tuna) and a wholegrain such as barley or brown rice for a balanced and colourful-looking meal.

Serves 2

Ingredients

50g wholemeal breadcrumbs
2 garlic cloves, chopped
4 anchovy fillets, chopped (you can buy marinated anchovies at deli counters of some supermarkets)

1 handful of parsley, stalks removed
2 tablespoons sesame seeds
4 tablespoons hemp or flaxseed oil
2 tuna steaks, 125g each

Method

In a food processor, whizz together the breadcrumbs, garlic, anchovies, parsley and sesame seeds while drizzling in the oil to make a thick paste.

Grill or shallow fry the tuna for around 2–3 minutes each side. Don't overcook: the tuna steaks should be still pink in the centre.

Spoon the cold topping over the cooked tuna to serve.

Herrings on Rye

Pickled herrings are not only a very handy store-cupboard ingredient but also a great source of omega 3s. Bought vacuum-packed beetroot is easy to use and convenient and is a good antioxidant. I'm using butter to stick this sandwich together – yes, it's a saturated fat, but at least it is a natural fat.

Serves 1

Ingredients

2 large slices rye bread or pumpernickel

a smear of butter

1 beetroot, cooked, skinned and sliced

2 small sprigs of fresh dill

125g cured herrings

Method

Spread the bread with a thin smear of butter then top with the rest of the ingredients to make an open sandwich – the herring and beetroot will stick to bread and butter.

Salmon

Salmon is a great source of protein, potassium, selenium and vitamin B12. It is also a rich source of EPA and DHA which are then processed to make prostaglandin series 3 which is anti-inflammatory. Wild salmon is expensive and hard to buy, and also the quality will vary, whereas farmed salmon is a more reliable source. But a whole range of quality issues surround farmed salmon. Salmon should not be bright orange or excessively fatty. Cheaper farmed salmon is often fattened up on oil to make it heavier and yield a higher price. The fish may often have been fed dyed food to make it appear more 'salmon' coloured. It is definitely worth buying organic farmed salmon or salmon from a farmer who can be seen to have made an effort to farm the fish to the highest standards. Smoked salmon usually involves brining the fish, then smoking over wood to preserve the fish, and should not affect the quality of the omega 3 fatty acids.

Zingy Warm Salmon Salad

This is a fantastic way to eat salmon and enjoy those wonderful omega 3-rich oils. This Vietnamese-inspired dish is adapted from a recipe by Australian chef Jill Dupleix and the fresh herbs, lime and chilli give it a real zing. Fish sauce is made from fermented fish – don't smell it, just use it as a great way to add salt and body to a host of dishes.

Serves 4

Ingredients

Sauce

150g soft, light brown sugar
150ml water

3 cloves garlic, chopped
4 tablespoons fish sauce

1 red chilli, deseeded and
   sliced
knob of ginger, peeled and sliced

4 tablespoons fresh lime
   juice

Salmon Salad

200g beansprouts
500g salmon fillets, cut in chunks
2 tablespoons vegetable oil
handful fresh mint leaves,
   chopped

handful fresh coriander
   leaves, chopped
1 spring onion, finely
   chopped
100g roasted salted
   peanuts, crushed

Method

First make the sauce. Put the sugar and water in a small pan and bring to the boil. Add the chilli, ginger and garlic and simmer till you have a rich, syrupy sauce (about 10 minutes). Remove from the heat, sieve and add the fish sauce and lime juice to the smooth sauce.

Next, pour boiling water over the beansprouts, leave for about 30 seconds, then drain and set aside.

To cook the salmon, heat the oil in a frying pan, pour a little of the sauce onto the salmon and stir-fry till cooked but still moist and tender. Take off the heat.

In a big bowl, toss the salmon with the mint, coriander, spring onion, peanuts, drained beansprouts and the rest of the warm sauce.

Herring in Oatmeal

When we filmed *The Woman Who Ate Scotland* on the north-west coast of Scotland it was raining and dark when I finally arrived at the Plockton Hotel. The hotel's chef, Alan Pearson, showed me how to make this traditional Scottish dish which has remained popular throughout the centuries. This delicious, fast-food fish dish is very good for you as herring and oats – Alan used fresh, local ingredients – are rich in essential fatty acids, good for the joints and for the brain. He recommends that no salt should be used when cooking fish as it is naturally salty.

Serves 4

Ingredients

2 tablespoons plain flour
2 eggs, beaten with
  50ml milk
200g pinhead oatmeal mixed
  with 50g fine oatmeal

4 herring fillets, skin on
25g unsalted butter
150ml vegetable oil
parsley and lemon wedges
  to garnish

Method

Sift the flour onto a flat plate, pour the egg and milk into a shallow bowl, and spread the oatmeal on a flat plate. Dip both sides of each herring fillet in the flour, then into the egg and milk and then into the oatmeal.

Put the butter and oil into a frying pan and turn up the heat till the butter starts to brown. Lay the herrings in the pan, skin side down first and fry for a couple of minutes on each side.

Serve flesh side up and garnished with parsley and lemon.

Omega 3s and meat

I was giving a small food demo extolling the joys of omega 3 at the Taste of Edinburgh Food Festival and I had set up a tasting of hot and cold smoked salmon. Nearby was a beef farmer from the Borders who must have been fuming at my suggestion that oily fish alone were a great source of omega 3s. He came over and told me about his cows which are fed on grass as opposed to all grain, and that his beef was therefore a good source of omega 3s. The omega 3s end up in the beef in the same way as the flesh of fish eating omega 3-rich plankton. Hens fed on an omega 3-rich diet will lay omega 3-rich eggs and their meat should also be a source of omega 3s.

It is getting easier to buy grass-fed beef, pork and lamb. As a result of being fed grass and having to work for their food, the cattle are leaner and do not have a lot of spare fat, so their beef has less saturated fat. But be very careful not to overcook: grass-fed beef needs about thirty per cent less cooking time than most common beef and is best if cooked medium-rare to medium, or it will be too tough. But on the other hand it has a different flavour – purists would say how beef used to taste! So it's worth seeking out grass-fed meat if possible for health and taste reasons.

Omega 3 Beef Burger with Caramelised Onions

The meat from grass-fed cattle is generally 80–90 per cent leaner than grain fed so, to add a bit of extra juice, these hamburgers are best served with caramelised onions – or, perhaps, a salsa.

Serves 1

Ingredients

25g unsalted butter

1 tablespoon olive oil

1 onion, finely sliced

2 tablespoons soft brown sugar

½ tablespoon red wine vinegar

sea salt and freshly ground black pepper

100g minced beef from grass-fed cattle

1 wholemeal roll

Method

Heat the butter and oil in a small frying pan. When hot, add the sliced onion and fry till it becomes a lovely gooey mass (about 20 minutes). Add the sugar and cook until the onions caramelise. Stir in the vinegar and season with salt and pepper.

While the onions are cooking shape your burger into a 2cm thick, 12cm round, with a small depression in the centre.

Preheat the grill to its hottest. Beef from grass-fed cattle cooks quicker than other beef, so grill for only about 2 minutes on one side and 3 on the other. Don't press on the burger as it cooks, you'll lose the delicious juices.

Remove the burger from the grill and let it rest for

about 5 minutes – this helps redistribute the juices throughout the meat so that it retains as much moisture as possible.

Split the roll and lay the cut halves on the grill to lightly toast. Serve the burger topped with caramelised onions inside the roll.

South-East Asian Anti-Inflammatory Rice Salad

This dish harnesses so many of the anti-inflammatory elements in food – sesame oil, omega oils, garlic, pineapple and sesame seeds – and is a lovely quick meal that can be eaten warm, straight from the pot. You can also chill and eat the next day, or enjoy as a packed lunch. This is a great way to use up extra rice.

Serves 2–3

Ingredients

250g brown rice
2 tablespoons sesame oil
5 tablespoons flaxseed
    or hemp oil
juice of 1 orange
2 cloves garlic, finely chopped
1 teaspoon sea salt
2 tablespoons soy sauce
2 tablespoons cider vinegar
1 pineapple, peeled and
    chopped

1 red pepper, finely chopped
1 small onion, finely chopped
225g can water chestnuts,
    drained
75g cashew nuts or roasted
    soybeans
75g raisins
2 tablespoons sesame seeds

Method

Cook the rice in boiling water until *al dente*: this can take 15–30 minutes depending on the type of brown rice.

Meanwhile, prepare the salad. Combine the sesame oil, omega oil, orange juice, garlic, salt, soy sauce and cider vinegar in a bowl. Add these ingredients to the cooked, rinsed rice while it's still warm.

Then add the chopped pineapple, red pepper, onion, water chestnuts, cashew nuts or soybeans, raisins and sesame seeds and mix through before serving.

Kind to your Knees Cherry Clafoutis

Cherries have anti-inflammatory properties so this is a great all-year-round traditional French dessert. I wish I had known about the healing powers of cherry clafoutis when I was stuck up the mountain all those years ago!

Serves 4

Ingredients

500g fresh cherries or
    425g can of stoned
    cherries in syrup
250ml semi-skimmed milk or
    soya milk

3 eggs
75g wholemeal or soya flour
50g soft brown brown sugar
1 teaspoon vanilla extract
icing sugar

Method

Preheat the oven to 200°C/400°F/Gas 6.

Arrange the cherries over a greased 25cm round baking dish.

In a food processor, or by hand, beat the milk and eggs together then gradually add the flour, sugar and vanilla extract to make a smooth batter.

Pour the batter over the fruit and bake for 20 minutes until just set and golden brown. Dust with icing sugar and serve warm or cold.

Anti-inflammatory Checklist

- EFAs – eat lots of oily fish, nuts and seeds and nut and seed oils.
- Lots of green vegetables and pulses maintain an alkaline balance in the body.
- Lots of squash, broccoli, kale and dark berries help with production of good prostaglandins.
- Ginger and turmeric have anti-inflammatory properties as do cherries and fresh pineapple.
- Avoid junk, processed or refined carbohydrate foods.
- Avoid foods made with trans and saturated fats.
- Avoid foods high in wheat and sugar.
- Avocados, sesame seeds, pumpkin seeds and sunflower seeds are all rich in vitamin E which can calm inflammation.

Have a Good Anti-inflammatory Day!

Breakfast: quinoa porridge with two teaspoons soaked linseeds and fresh pineapple, so some protein with lots of omega 3, and bromelian or pumpkin seed butter on rye toast.

Snack: handful of baked soya beans which are a good source of omega 6.

Lunch: oatcakes, beetroot and pickled herring; more omega 3 from the herring.

Snack: strawberry or berry yoghurt smoothie with omega oil balance of omega 3 and 6.

Evening meal: veggie moussaka and chopped avocado and green salad dressed with hemp seed oil – lots of alkaline vegetables and anti-inflammatory spices as well as omegas 3 and 6 from oil dressing.

Water: Drink one and a half litres of water.

Exercise: thirty minutes gentle exercise boosts circulation, eases stress and helps get oxygen and oils round your body.

Bonuses: as well as fewer aches and pains, glossy hair, clear skin, strong nails, good mood with fewer mood swings; feel mentally on the ball, as all these good omegas benefit the brain; plus lowered blood pressure and better heart health.

How to Have a Happy, Healthy Digestive System

7

One in three people suffer from Irritable Bowel Syndrome (IBS) and undiagnosed bowel problems, and yet there is very little publicity about it; no one does sponsored walks in aid of it, or holds charity concerts and most of the one in three find it embarrassing to explain to people that they suffer from bouts of crippling constipation, got-to-go-diarrhoea, uncomfortable bloating, noxious wind and painful abdominal cramps. These symptoms all fall under the umbrella name of IBS. If you suffer from any of them, I hope this chapter will help with explaining why you might be suffering and what you can do to ease the symptoms by eating the right kind of balanced varied diet.

IBS is actually quite a vague name; irritable in this context means inflamed, your bowel is part of your digestive tract which runs from your mouth to your anus, and syndrome in medical terms means a collection of symptoms. IBS is classified as a functional disorder; there is no clinical explanation of why people should repeatedly suffer from either or all of these digestive disorders, or just one of them, but addressing diet and lifestyle can be a very effective solution in treating recurrent constipation, diarrhoea and wind.

There is no test for IBS, as on examination the bowels have no perceivable damage or irritation; the only signs are the symptoms, which to a patient are very real. Doctors usually diagnose IBS if you have been suffering from a combination of recurring constipation, diarrhoea, bloating and/or excess wind on and off for more than twelve weeks. This seems like a long time to be toilet-centric, but there are wide parameters for 'normal' bowel movements. Stools the consistency of rabbit droppings and watery stools are not normal. What you are looking for is something in between and here one can get quite graphic or quite lyrical. I saw an advert on television once for a laxative, with the tag line 'the joy of movement'. I think it would be a good goal to aim to pass a comfortable, 'joyous' stool at least once a day, to keep ridding your body of toxic waste.

Your bowel is very sensitive, has numerous nerve endings and responds very quickly to your emotions and hormones; it is perfectly normal to experience a difference in bowel habits if you alter your diet, lifestyle, routine, go on holiday, exercise more, are stressed at work or go through relationship ups and downs – all these will be mirrored in your bowel movements. This again makes it hard for doctors to pinpoint what causes the large intestine either to slow down its contractions – to expel the waste (constipation) – or speed up the contractions in an irritated way (diarrhoea). These spasms can also cause abdominal cramps, and irregular contractions cause build up of gas.

But first it is important to establish whether or not you have IBS. If there is any significant change in your bowel movements, weight loss, or a fever and especially if any blood is passed, it is worth getting a doctor to rule out anything more seriously wrong such as ulcerative colitis (inflammation and ulcers in the large intestine); Crohn's disease (inflammation of any part of the digestive tract and its deeper layers); diverticulosis (the bowel's mucous lining breaks through the outer muscle layers causing pouches on the bowel wall) or even bowel cancer. These diseases share some of the symptoms of IBS, but tend not to disappear and reappear. There are tests for these diseases, so it is better to let a doctor decide whether or not you have IBS, rather than begin self-medicating.

You don't have to live with diarrhoea, constipation and wind. It can have knock-on effects; repeated straining to pass stools can damage the veins round the anus (haemorrhoids) which may then become painful. If they don't heal you may need medical attention. IBS can also cause tiredness (lack of nutrients being absorbed), lethargy, back pain and make sexual intercourse painful, which can all lead to anxiety and depression, so don't suffer, you can control IBS and the best way is through eating well.

Understanding Your Bowel

Digestion starts in the mouth where simple carbohydrates are broken down into sugars, then continues on in the stomach where proteins are mainly digested, then through rhythmic contractions your stomach expels this mush of partially digested food into the small intestine where digestion of

most of the fats, carbo-
hydrates, the rest of the
protein, vitamins and minerals takes place, and the
nutrients absorbed. The
leftover is mainly waste

Good bacteria also support your immune system

which passes into the large intestine or colon where water and
salts are absorbed. By this time it should be a soft solid
material ready to be expelled. Good bacteria live in both
intestines and they can play a huge part in helping to break
down food and aid absorption. In the small intestine they help
with absorption and also make certain vitamins, while in the
large intestine they are involved in eliminating waste. Good
bacteria also support your immune system.

No one knows exactly what causes IBS or what makes the
bowel irritated, but usually there is a trigger:

- Gastrointestinal infection – if you have had a bug, then even
  though you have got over the worst of it, new bacteria may
  have upset the balance of good and bad bacteria in the
  small intestine.
- Antibiotics – IBS symptoms can flare up after a course of
  antibiotics as they have wiped out all the good bacteria in
  the small intestine.
- You may have been on holiday or even closer to home and
  picked up a parasite which will cause IBS symptoms, mainly
  bloating, very smelly wind, lethargy and watery stools. A
  stool test can confirm presence of parasites.
- Periods of anxiety or stress – remember Chapter Four,
  Coping With Stress? Powerful hormones adrenalin and
  cortisol are released in response to stress and they can have
  their effect on the bowel. In times of stress, blood is diverted

away from the stomach and intestines to the brain and muscles, so digestion is often slowed down and impaired.

- Hormones – for women oestrogen and progesterone levels vary at different times of their menstrual cycle. Progesterone slows down the rate of movement in the large intestine which can lead to constipation. Progesterone levels rise in the second half of your menstrual cycle as your body is preparing itself for potential pregnancy. This might explain why pregnant women are prone to constipation, as there are higher levels of progesterone in their blood.

Consider these triggers if you have suddenly started experiencing digestive problems, but also look at your diet; the primary cause of IBS is diet. The main problems (constipation, diarrhoea and wind) associated with IBS occur in the large intestine. The large intestine's function is to absorb water back into the body and get rid of the waste products of digestion as regularly and efficiently as possible. Your intestine likes fibre as fibre helps move the mass along. Fibre also promotes the presence of healthy gut bacteria, helps lower cholesterol and slows down glucose absorption in your bloodstream, thus regulating blood glucose. It also absorbs any excess oestrogen – a lack of fibre means oestrogen gets reabsorbed. This can be linked with cancers that affect the reproductive organs.

Fibre

Dietary fibre is found in plants: cereals, pulses, fruits and vegetables. Meat and fish have very little fibre. Fibre is found in the cell walls of edible plant tissue and in the seeds of certain plants. But there is more to fibre than just 'eating your greens and being done with it' – there are two kinds of fibre: insoluble and soluble, and you need a balance of them both for healthy, enjoyable 'joy of movement' bowel actions. Fibre cannot be broken down by human digestive enzymes, so it passes through the stomach and its acids relatively unscathed, until it reaches the intestines where bacteria which inhabit the intestine are able to start to break the fibre down producing gases (carbon dioxide, methane and hydrogen) and short chain fatty acids which are absorbed into the cells of the gut wall for energy or passed on into the bloodstream.

Soluble Fibre Soluble means it dissolves in water, a type of fibre broken down by enzyme-producing bacteria through the process of fermentation in the small intestine to produce energy and gas. Soluble fibre needs water and forms a gel-like substance which is smooth and soothing to the gut. It can also bind to other substances such as cholesterol and hormones. Oats lower cholesterol, as the soluble fibre in the oats binds up the cholesterol and carries it out of the body as waste. Soluble fibre also helps slow down blood sugar into the bloodstream.

Most plant sources have a mix of soluble and insoluble fibre. Good sources of predominantly soluble fibre are:

- Most fruits
- Most vegetables
- Barley
- Oats
- Pulses – beans and lentils
- Seeds

Insoluble Fibre Insoluble means that the fibre won't dissolve in water and is less easily broken down by the intestinal bacteria than soluble fibre. But it attracts water so it can help to increase bulk, soften stools and shorten food transit time through your intestinal tract. This increased bulk gives your muscle walls something to contract against and help push the waste material towards your anus for expulsion.

Sources of predominantly insoluble fibre include:

- Fruits and vegetables with skins, husks and skins
- Wholegrain foods such as wholewheat, spelt, buckwheat, millet, brown rice
- Chickpeas
- Rye
- Wheat
- Soybeans
- Vegetables such as green beans, sweetcorn, cauliflower, celery and vegetables with skins like peas and broad beans
- Almonds
- Oat bran

Wheat bran can ease constipation as it leads to bulkier stools, but it is still derived from wheat, which could irritate if you are intolerant. It is also quite coarse and can irritate an already sensitive bowel; oat bran or psyllium husks are gentler.

You require about one third insoluble fibre to two thirds soluble fibre in your diet for optimum bowel movement, but it is not as complicated as it seems. Eat the whole apple – not the core unless you like it, but the skin as well – and you will get the right balance (be sure to wash the skin first to remove dirt and any fungicide sprays).

You'll know if you are getting it right; too much soluble fibre and you get a stool that is soft and ribbon like and hard to push, as there is no bulk to push against the bowel wall and make the muscle contract naturally, while too much insoluble fibre could cause bloating and wind. Fibre is also very dependent on water. The recommended amount hovers round the one and a half litre mark, but let your body tell you. Once again, if you have dark urine, you need to drink more water. You are aiming for pale yellow urine. It's worth remembering if you are eating more vegetables that they are full of water, so it's not just about counting glasses of water, but being aware of how much you need to drink – if you feel thirsty, you are dehydrated.

As well as enjoying a pleasurable toilet experience, you will also benefit from eating fibre because it:

- Lowers blood cholesterol levels.
- Helps to remove excess hormones and toxins from your body
- Helps to control blood glucose levels – so very good if you are concerned with weight loss and diabetes

You might be ready for a change of eating pattern, but your bowel might not be. Like any muscle in your body which has not been used, you need to introduce it to work gradually. After a diet high in processed foods with little fibre your bowel muscles may not have had to work very hard. Increase both kind of fibres gradually until you have a bowel movement you enjoy, perhaps by adding a couple of tablespoons of lentils to white rice, or by mixing brown and white rice.

If you like processed wheat pasta don't suddenly change overnight; mix wholemeal pasta with your usual pasta, until your taste buds and your bowel muscles adapt. Try to make sure you are eating a mix of soluble and insoluble fibre – the easiest way is to eat washed unpeeled fruit and vegetables and veggie stews with a wholegrain of pulse. Remember that transit time – from the moment you put the food in your mouth, to when the waste is expelled as faeces – varies from about eighteen to thirty-six hours, so be patient and don't expect to see results overnight.

How Much Fibre Do You Need?

The average fibre intake in Britain is 12g per day. The Food Standard Agency recommends that it should be 18g per day for adults, and maximum of 30g. According to their recommendations a 'source' of fibre should contain 3g per 100g (or per 100ml). For a claim of high fibre the food must contain at least 6g per 100g (or per 100ml) so it is interesting to look at the back of food packets. For example, a commercial muesli containing wheat and rye flakes, dried fruit, almonds and seeds has a fibre component of 7.6g per 100g recommended serving, so it deserves to call itself high fibre. Wholemeal bread has 8.1g of fibre per 100g whereas sliced white comes in at 2.4g per 100g . A rough oatcake has 5.6g per 100g, but a digestive biscuit has 2.9g per 100g and will also have higher amounts of saturated fat and sugar. Normal supermarket pasta has 3g of fibre per 100g, while wholemeal has 9g per 100g.

Food Intolerances

Certain foods can trigger IBS symptoms; an enzyme or chemical can irritate the bowel wall which can cause constipation or diarrhoea or abdominal cramps. You can get blood tests, but they are not always accurate and can only measure what enzymes are in your blood at that precise moment. These can fluctuate and your reaction can change too over time, so be wary of ruling food outs. A more dependable but boring route – no exciting Eureka moments – is by cutting out certain foods and reintroducing them after a few weeks, then recording the differences and getting to know your own body and how it reacts. The way to do this is by keeping a food diary. Every day, list what you ate, drank, your bowel movements and mood, then you will have more chance of spotting foods that may be irritating your bowels. The goal is to avoid these foods, for a couple of weeks, then gradually re-introduce. The mission is to achieve a balanced diet with as few foods removed as possible.

There are certain suspect foods which crop up time and time again and it is worth being aware of them:

- Wheat can irritate your bowel on several counts. First of all it contains gluten which is a protein made up of two smaller proteins – glutenin and gliadin – which can irritate the gut wall, and in the case of coeliacs trigger an immune response to attack the lining of the gut wall. Coeliac disease is relatively rare and can be confirmed with a blood test. Rye, barley and oats both contain gluten but the proteins are configured slightly differently, so they do not always irritate. Second, wheat is very processed now, so it lacks any kind of fibre and the cheapest most processed forms will turn to sticky wallpaper paste in your gut. So opt for more complex wheat grain such as spelt which is the original form of the grain before it became over-processed.

- Caffeine-containing foods and drinks as caffeine stimulate the bowel wall.

- Dairy products – milk, cheese, ice cream. For some people it can be an intolerance to the milk sugar lactose – if you don't have enough of the enzyme lactase to digest the lactose sugars in milk; you can be tested for lactose intolerance. There is often no need to cut dairy out completely, but have a little as part of a meal. The fermentation process of yoghurt means that most of the lactose has been broken down by the good bacteria, so yoghurt is less likely to cause upset and in fact is good for encouraging growth of good bacteria in the small intestine.

- Fruit juices – they are acidic and also contain fructose, a fruit sugar which can irritate the intestine wall in the same way as lactose.
- Additives and preservatives used in food such as sulphur dioxide.
- Artificial sweeteners. Many low-carbohydrate diet foods are sweetened with lacitol or sorbitol, which are sugar alcohols, and, when eaten in large quantities, can cause digestive disturbances.

Balance

It's not a case of never eating these foods, just of being careful and reading the small print on the back of packets. I love dried apricots and when I was working as an editor of a food magazine I commissioned a story on Yin and Yang foods, drawing on the Chinese philosophy on achieving balance. Yang foods are believed to increase the body's heat (raise the metabolic rate), while Yin foods are believed to decrease the body's heat (lower the metabolic rate). The Chinese ideal is to eat both types of food to keep the body in balance. To illustrate the article the food stylist made a lovely yin yang collage out of golden fat apricots and contrasting dark brown lentils which we photographed for the article.

Afterwards I wolfed down all these left-over apricots – but of course it is all a question of balance – and I suffered the most incredible abdominal cramps while playing squash. They were so bad I remember lying on the court in agony waiting for the spasms to pass. Then rather unfairly to apricots, I avoided them until I was cycling with a group of friends in Pakistan. We had come over the 5,000-metre Kunjerab Pass from Western China, a desolate area where there is very little food – one night we even resorted to eating vitamin tablets boiled in rice – to the very rich fertile Hunza Valley in Pakistan. We were cycling in the peak of apricot season, and as we rounded a corner before us was a horizon of vivid orange coloured roof-tops: fresh apricots drying in the hot sun.

These dried apricots were like nothing I had tasted before; they were concentrated golden nectar and I bought bagfuls of them thinking: 'I don't care about the consequences, they are worth it.' But despite my insouciant gluttony, I did not suffer one spasm of pain. I think it was the sulphur dioxide used to dry the more cosmetically attractive apricots that had caused my abdominal cramps, not the apricots themselves. Try to buy naturally dried apricots, they are not so cosmetically attractive and are wizened, but are packed with more flavour and less likely to cause bowel reaction. Check the label to see if sulphur dioxide has been used to dry the fruit. Also be aware that most wines are finished with sulphites. It usually warns you on the label – and this could be a reason why you have a headache or stomach ache the next morning!

The Way Forward

You need to get your bowel contractions back to a normal pace, not too fast (diarrhoea) or too slow (constipation) so you are aiming for a balanced diet of protein, complex carbohydrates, soluble and insoluble fibre and unsaturated fat at each meal.

Guidelines for IBS sufferers:

- Eat regular but small meals/snacks – this is easier for your digestive system.
- Make lunch your main meal and don't have a late evening meal, so your body can finish digesting before you go to bed.
- Chew well.
- Don't rush eating, sit down and enjoy, make time to eat.
- Don't eat sugary processed foods as high blood sugar can decrease intestinal motility and even stop it completely. Also excessive sugar changes the environment in the intestines, making it less favourable for good bacteria to thrive.
- Avoid saturated fats, wheatbran, dairy, red meat, alcohol, caffeine and spices. Avoiding dairy is an understandable concern as you risk missing out on calcium, but good sources of calcium – and magnesium which you need to uptake calcium – are found in green vegetables, broccoli, kale and olives, figs, apricots, dates, hazelnuts, almonds, brazil nuts and small fish with bones such as anchovies as well as tofu.

> Don't rush eating, sit down and enjoy, make time to eat

IBS can manifest itself as a combination of diarrhoea, constipation or a mixture of both. If your IBS takes the form of diarrhoea, then you need to encourage your bowel not to keep emptying so often and reintroduce fibrous foods gradually. During or after an attack:

- Eat stewed peeled fruit and lightly cooked vegetables with no skin.
- Eat white fish, avoid oily fish as it is harder to digest.

- Enjoy non-gluten grains; rice, quinoa, then gradually introduce more wholegrains.
- Drink water to replace the extra lost through the bowel. After a bout of diarrhoea you will have also lost salts so a natural way is to replace them by eating a bowl of vegetable soup.
- Eat pectin-rich fruits such as pears, and apples; they can help form a comforting gel in the intestine (pectin helps jam to set) and tannin-rich, stool-firming blueberries.

If your IBS takes the form of constipation, then you need to encourage the bowel to speed up its contractions and again reintroduce fibrous foods gradually.

- Focus on complex carbohydrates which tend to have soluble and insoluble fibre – see introduction on complex carbohydrates; variety is important, so experiment with different grains.
- Your bowel may have become lazy, especially if you have been taking laxatives, so introduce both types of fibre gradually so it relearns to contract by itself. Add a tablespoon of cooked tinned puy lentils to a salad. Add a few tablespoons of red lentils to a vegetable soup. Make your own hummus from tinned chickpeas to use as a spread or a dip, again chickpeas are great for bulking up salads, soups and mild veggie curries.
- Remember to increase your water to cope with increasing amounts of fibre, otherwise constipation will worsen.
- Reduce caffeine or cut it out.
- Aloe vera is good for healing the gut and is a natural laxative, as are soaked linseeds.
- Gentle exercise can stimulate the bowels into action.
- Never put off bowel movements – as it means your intestines absorb more water, and stools become harder.

Wind/Flatulence

Some foods are more prone to causing wind than others. Pulses such as lentils and beans contain oligosaccharides – glucose molecules which your digestive system can't break down until they reach the intestines, where bacteria do eventually break them down, releasing wind. Cucumbers, onions, cabbage and Brussels sprouts, and other members of the brassica family, can also cause excess wind to be produced in your intestines due to their sulphur make-up. Jerusalem artichokes are notorious because they are made up of the starch inulin which, while promoting the growth of good bacteria in the small intestine, also causes wind. So enjoy them in small amounts. But your bowel can get used to processing these foods, so it is good to gradually introduce them into your diet.

Reducing wind:

- Too much soluble fibre can result in smelly wind; eat a counter balance of insoluble fibre. Oats are a great source of soluble fibre, but it is easy to think you are doing the right thing and adding them to everything from smoothies, to flapjacks to fruit crumbles. Don't go overboard on the oats, remember don't exceed 30g of fibre a day (jumbo oats contain 9g of fibre per 100g). Most carbohydrates can produce gas when broken down in your intestine. If that is a problem eat more rice which does not seem to produce excess gas.

- Enjoy natural live yoghurt – see Chapter Three for boosting immune recipes. Good bacteria in the intestine are affected by diarrhoea, stress and diet. These good bacteria colonise the large intestine particularly because the gut contents slow down dramatically when they reach the colon and because acidity levels are lower. They stimulate your immune system, kill off disease-causing organisms and also make some B vitamins. Probiotics can reduce gas formation in the bowel and thus minimise bloating. They also increase resistance to food poisoning and can prevent diarrhoea associated with antibiotic use. These wonder bacteria can also reduce cholesterol levels and can help heal damage and inflammation in your gut wall.

- Eat low GI fruit – cherries, pears and apples rather than grapes or melon which are so high in simple sugars that they can ferment in the intestines with foods eaten later.
- Eat slowly, so you don't gulp and cause wind that way.
- Drink herbal teas such as peppermint, chamomile and fennel. Fresh ginger is a carminative (something which promotes the elimination of intestinal wind and also relaxes and soothes the intestinal tract). Chop and add to hot water. Fresh dill added to boiling water and strained after five minutes can help reduce wind – sip throughout day. Also a good way to avoid wind is to make sure you are drinking enough water, so herbal teas have a dual purpose.

Recipes

These are all geared for good all-round bowel health, but are delicious in their own right, so enjoy and also mix and match flavours and textures to suit yourself.

Breakfast

As always, it is good to start the day with breakfast for energy, blood sugar management and to provide something for the bowels to work with. Oats are a great soluble fibre, so porridge and muesli are good fibre-building starts to the day. Even better to add some rye flakes which are a good source of insoluble fibre as they bind with water in your intestinal tract, so you feel full and are less tempted to hit the mid-morning muffin later.

Make-your-Own Almond and Cranberry Muesli

This is a handy mixture of soluble and insoluble fibre. The beauty of making your own muesli is you can tailor it to your taste.

When buying oats choose unflattened kernels or steel-cut oats, which are cut quickly by steel blades to give a dense, chewy texture.

I like to soak my muesli in fruit juice, such as freshly squeezed apple or orange – this helps to make it more easily digestible. I also add two teaspoonfuls of linseeds soaked in warm water till they swell. If linseeds are not soaked your body can't break down the outer seed shell and you will miss out on their omega 3s as well as their fibre; alternatively, you can crack the seeds using a pestle and mortar.

Makes 4–6 servings of muesli

Ingredients

200g oats
1 tablespoon rye flakes
1 tablespoon oat bran
1 tablespoon wheat germ
75g whole almonds,
  chopped

50g dried cranberries
2 tablespoons sunflower seeds
2 tablespoons pumpkin seeds
fruit juice, probiotic yoghurt,
  soaked or cracked linseeds
  and/or honey to serve

Method

Mix all the ingredients together up to and including the pumpkin seeds in a large bowl. Store for up to a month in an airtight container. Feel free to vary amounts and ingredients.

To serve, soak in fruit juice for about 10 minutes, add soaked or cracked linseeds and top with probiotic yoghurt and a spoonful of honey.

Rye Bread with Figs and Pecans

This bread is quite solid, but comes into its own when toasted. Figs are also a good source of fibre and pecans bump up the protein.

Rye grains look like wheat grains, but they are harder to process, so rye flour still contains most of its nutrient and fibre. Rye's gluten is less elastic than that of wheat, it does not rise so much when baked and, thus, makes for a dense bread.

Rye also has lots of non-cellulose polysaccharides which have a high water-binding capacity – so you'll feel full.

Ingredients

300g rye flour
200g wholemeal flour
100g dried figs, chopped
50g pecan nuts, chopped

7g dried yeast
1 teaspoon soft brown sugar
1 teaspoon sea salt
200ml warm water

Method

Preheat the oven to 180°C/350°F/Gas 4.

Put all the dry ingredients in a bowl, add the warm water and mix to a sticky dough. Turn out onto a floured surface and knead till smooth.

Put the pliable dough in a greased, 23x13cm loaf tin with room for the dough to almost double in height and leave for about an hour to rise.

Bake for about 40 minutes. Allow to cool then slice. The bread freezes well – freeze in slices, so easy to toast straight from the freezer.

Kedgeree

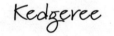

This is a good breakfast or supper meal which is a valuable source of soluble fibre from the red lentils and insoluble from the brown rice – it even looks pretty with flecks of fresh coriander and yellow-yolked boiled egg.

The spices add flavour, but reduce or omit them to suit your taste.

Serves 2

Ingredients

150g undyed smoked haddock

100ml milk, enough to cover fish

100g short-grain or long-grain brown rice

2 eggs

100g red lentils

300ml hot water

1–2 teaspoons ground coriander

1–2 teaspoons ground cumin

20g fresh coriander, stalks removed and chopped

Method

Poach the haddock in just enough milk for about 5 minutes – till cooked through but still moist – drain (reserve the juices) and set aside.

Put the rice in boiling water and cook till tender, drain and set aside.

Soft-boil the eggs for 4 minutes, peel, slice and set aside.

In a separate pan, simmer the lentils in water, with the coriander and cumin, until soft.

Mix together the rice and lentils. Flake in the haddock, along with some reserved juices to the rice/lentil mix, stir in the coriander and top with egg.

Soups

Soups are a great way to increase liquid and electrolytes into your diet. You are also in control of the fibre; you can thicken by adding chickpeas or lentils to the cooking liquid or enjoy soup with a slice of wholemeal bread. Also if you want less fibre, peel vegetables and use fewer vegetables, so you are basically just enjoying a stock. Organic stock cubes are best, as some of the more commercial may have intestinal irritants. Or splash out and buy good quality liquid stock.

Restorative Carrot, Orange and Ginger Soup

Carrot soup provides a good source of soluble fibre. This gentle soup is ideal if you are suffering from diarrhoea and want to avoid irritating your bowel with too much insoluble fibre.

The orange brings vitamin C to the party and fresh ginger may have anti-inflammatory properties and can reduce flatulence.

Serve with oatcakes or wholemeal bread if you're looking to bulk things up.

Serves 2

Ingredients

1 tablespoon vegetable oil

1 onion, chopped

4 carrots, peeled and chopped (remove the hard woody core to avoid insoluble fibre)

knob of fresh ginger, peeled and chopped

500ml vegetable stock, made with non-additive cubes such as Kallo organic or Marigold Swiss Bouillon powder

juice of 1 orange

sea salt and freshly ground pepper

Method

In a large pot, heat the oil and gently cook the onion till soft. Add the chopped carrots, ginger and hot stock and simmer till the carrots soften (about 15 minutes).

Blend in a food processor (or use a hand blender in the pan), add the orange juice and season with salt and pepper.

Green-for-Go Pea and Mint Soup

This is a very easy soup to make and most of the ingredients are store cupboard/freezer material – ideal if you're not in the mood for shopping.

Peas are a good source of soluble and insoluble fibre – think of all the skin around each little pea.

Serves 2

Ingredients

1 tablespoon vegetable oil
1 onion, chopped
400g frozen peas
600ml vegetable stock, made
   with non-additive cubes such
   as Kallo organic or Marigold
   Swiss Bouillon powder

handful of fresh mint leaves,
   roughly chopped (keep
   2 sprigs for garnish)
yoghurt to serve

Method

In a large pot, heat the oil and gently cook the onions till soft. Add the frozen peas and hot stock then simmer for about 5 minutes. Tip into a food processor, add the fresh mint and blend (or use a hand blender in the pot).

To serve, garnish with a swirl of yoghurt and a sprig of mint – it's important to keep up standards even when you're feeling under the weather.

Fennel Soup

Fennel belongs to the same family as celery and carrot and it has a lovely, aniseed flavour. Fennel can also help to dispel flatulence and it may ease intestinal spasms and inflammation, so it can be beneficial for those with irritable bowel syndrome (IBS).

Serves 2

Ingredients

1 tablespoon olive oil

1 large fennel bulb, trimmed and sliced

2 cloves garlic, chopped

3 tablespoons parsley, stalks removed and chopped

600ml vegetable stock, made with non-additive cubes such as Kallo organic or Marigold Swiss Bouillon powder

Method

In a large pot, heat the oil, stir-fry the fennel then add the garlic and 2 tablespoons of the parsley. Pour in the hot stock and simmer till the fennel is very soft (about 40 minutes).

Add the remaining parsley, stir and serve. If you want a smoother soup, process in a blender.

Apricot and Lentil Soup

This is a delicious, filling, high-fibre soup. It's very good, but be wary of seconds until your intestines are used to pulses and dried fruit – this one's not for those still wearing their fibre L-plates.

Serves 2

Ingredients

1 tablespoon vegetable oil
1 onion, chopped
100g red lentils
75g unsulphured apricots,
   chopped

500ml vegetable stock, made
   with non-additive cubes such as
   Kallo organic or Marigold Swiss
   Bouillon powder
sea salt and freshly ground
   pepper (optional)

Method

In a large pot, heat the oil and gently cook the onion till soft. Add the lentils and dried apricots and stir for a few minutes then add the hot stock and simmer till the lentils and apricots soften (about 20 minutes). Tip into a food processor and whizz (or use a hand blender in the pot).

Season if you wish with salt and pepper to taste.

Egyptian Rice and Lentil Stew

This is a popular Egyptian dish which I discovered when I was a member of the Arabic society at university – though I have to confess my interest was in food, not the Seven Pillars of Islam.

As well as being a good source of soluble and insoluble fibre this stew is also rich in complementary amino acids so it is a good veggie protein meal. If onions don't agree with you, omit or reduce the amount.

Serve with probiotic yoghurt.

Serves 4

Ingredients

125g red lentils
250g brown rice
2 tablespoons vegetable oil

2 large onions, sliced
salt and pepper, to season
probiotic yoghurt to serve

Method

Put the lentils in a pan with enough water to cover and cook until soft. In another pan, cook the rice.

While the lentils and rice are cooking, heat the oil in a frying pan and fry the onions till soft, golden and caramelised, taking care not to let them burn.

Mix the drained rice and lentils together with a little water and warm though. Season with salt and pepper.

Spread the lentil/rice mix over a large shallow dish and top with the fried onion slices and a dollop of yoghurt.

Chicken with Almonds and Prunes

Prunes have gained a reputation for – that horrible expression – 'keeping you regular' and they are, indeed, a good source of soluble and insoluble fibre. They add a delicious sweetness and richness to this chicken dish which is livened up by sweet, anti-inflammatory spices.

Serves 4

Ingredients

1 tablespoon sunflower oil
2 onions, sliced
1 clove garlic, chopped
1 teaspoon turmeric
1 teaspoon ground cinnamon
1 teaspoon ground ginger

4 chicken breasts, skin off, cubed
500ml chicken stock
250g juicy prunes, stones removed and roughly chopped
25g slivered almonds, toasted

Method

Heat the oil in a medium pan and cook the onions for about 5 minutes till soft. Add the garlic, spices and chicken then stir to coat evenly. Pour in the hot stock, bring to the boil then cover and simmer for 15 minutes, stirring occasionally.

Add the prunes and simmer, lid on, for a further 15 minutes. Remove the lid, stir well and continue to simmer for 10 minutes more, till the chicken and prunes are tender and the sauce has thickened slightly.

Transfer to a serving dish and sprinkle with the almonds.

Gentle Lentils

This is a nice soluble fibre dish. You could add 100g of frozen spinach towards the end of cooking, to bump up the fibre and vegetable count.

Serve the lentils with a grain of your choice. Depending how much fibre you feel up to, choose anything from comforting white rice to millet or brown rice if you feel you want more bulk. Pulses and grains contain complementary amino acids, so their addition makes this a nutritious protein meal.

You could also spoon over some probiotic yoghurt to help your intestines break down the lentils.

Serves 1–2

Ingredients

200g red lentils
juice of 1 lemon
1 tablespoon olive oil
2 teaspoons coriander seeds,
   ground in a pestle and mortar

1 teaspoon ground cumin
sea salt

Method

Cook the lentils in water for about 20 minutes till soft then drain. Return to the pot, add the lemon juice, olive oil, the ground coriander and cumin. Season to taste with salt then warm through gently for about 10 minutes.

Chickpea Crumble

This is a good source of soluble and insoluble fibre.
Serve with a rocket and vitamin E-rich avocado salad.

Serves 2

Ingredients

Chickpea Base

1 teaspoon vegetable oil
1 small onion, chopped
1 small red pepper, deseeded
   and chopped
2 carrots, chopped

200g can tomatoes
175g canned chickpeas,
   drained
pinch of ground cumin

Crumble Topping

100g wholemeal or brown
   rice flour
25g porridge oats

1 tablespoon pumpkin seeds
3 tablespoons olive oil

Method

Preheat the oven to 190°C/375°F/Gas 5.

In a medium-sized pan, heat the oil and cook the onion until soft. Add the pepper and carrots and stir-fry for about 5 minutes. Add the tomatoes, chickpeas and cumin and simmer gently for 15 minutes. Add a little water, so it does not catch. Set aside.

To make the crumble topping, combine all the dry ingredients in a large bowl then gradually add the oil, mixing with your fingers till the mix is the consistency of large breadcrumbs.

Spoon the chickpea mixture into an ovenproof dish, top with crumble and bake for 30 minutes.

Eat-your-Greens Couscous

This is a lovely summery and very quick-to-make dish using frozen, fibre-packed vegetables and couscous. What nicer way to eat your greens?

Serves 2–3

Ingredients

Couscous

½ teaspoon salt
500ml boiling water

200g barley or wheat couscous
3 tablespoons olive oil

Green Vegetables

500ml vegetable stock, made
   with non-additive cubes such
   as Kallo organic or Marigold
   Swiss Bouillon powder
4 spring onions, chopped
100g frozen broad beans
100g frozen peas

100g frozen soya beans
handful of parsley, leaves
   only, chopped
handful of coriander, leaves
   only, chopped
handful of mint, leaves
   only, chopped

Method

Dissolve the salt in the boiling water. Put the couscous in

a bowl, pour over enough water to cover, and let it sit for about 10 minutes till all the water has been absorbed. When the couscous has 'cooked', add the olive oil and gently fork it through to mix.

Meanwhile, put the hot stock in a large saucepan, bring to the boil, add the spring onions and all the frozen vegetables and simmer for 10 minutes. Just before serving add the fresh herbs and stir through.

Serve with the warm couscous in a pasta bowl, as it is quite liquidy.

Puds

It is always nice to finish with something sweet at the end of a meal, and stewed peeled fruit is gentle on a troubled digestive system. Pectin in pears and apples has a binding effect. Small fruits with skins still on, such as blackcurrants and blueberries, are good sources of soluble as well as insoluble fibre.

Comfort Is: Baked Apple Stuffed with Almonds and Dates

Apples are a good source of soluble fibre and rich in jam-setting pectin which is soothing for the gut. The almonds contain protein and are a source of insoluble fibre and the dates, too, add some fibre input.

Delicious hot or cold. This recipe serves one but just multiply the quantities to make more.

Serves 1

Ingredients

1 baking apple (such as
  Bramley)
2 tablespoons ground almonds
4–6 fresh dates, chopped

1 tablespoon clear honey
small knob of butter
4 tablespoons cold water

Method

Preheat the oven to 200°C/400°F/Gas 6.

Don't peel, but do wash and core the apple then cut a score around its 'equator' – so the skin can split while cooking.

In a small bowl, mix together the almonds, dates and honey to form a sticky paste.

Place the apple on a greased baking tray and stuff the empty core with the almond and date paste. Dot the butter on top of the paste.

Spoon 4 tablespoons water into the tray around the base of the apple and bake for 45–50 minutes till the flesh is tender and fluffy.

Spice-Roasted Fruits

Black pepper brings a richness and warmth to this spicy summer or winter fruit recipe – great hot or cold. Use any summer stone fruits – peaches, plums, nectarines etc. – and in winter, figs, pears etc.

It does not matter if the fruit is not fully ripe, the cooking makes it very edible.

Serves 4

Ingredients

2 cinnamon sticks, roughly broken up

4 star anise pods, broken to release oils

1 vanilla pod, seeds scraped

1 tablespoon clear honey

zest and juice of 1 orange

1 tablespoon soft brown sugar

½ teaspoon freshly ground black pepper

4–6 ripeish apricots

4–6 ripeish nectarines

20g unsalted butter

Method

Preheat the oven to 200°C/400°F/Gas 6.

In a small bowl, mix together the spices, vanilla, honey, orange zest and juice, sugar and pepper.

Stone and cut whichever fruit you are using in half and place it skin side down in a deep roasting dish.

Pour the spice mix all over the fruit, dot with the butter and bake for 45 minutes, basting occasionally.

Good Digestion Checklist

- Eat regular but small meals/snacks – this is easier for your digestive system.
- Include natural probiotic yoghurt in meals or as a snack.
- Make sure you include soluble and insoluble fibre in your diet – fruit, vegetables and pulses and lots of wholegrains.
- Drink enough water to counterbalance extra fibre in diet.
- Don't rush eating, sit down and enjoy, make time to eat.
- Don't eat sugary processed foods.

- Cut back on saturated fats, wheat bran, dairy, red meat, alcohol, caffeine and spices.
- Exercise can help digestion.

Have a Good Digestion Day!

Breakfast: toasted rye bread with pecan and figs and nut butter or ricotta cheese or kedgeree – a filling start to the day with good sources of fibre and fat and protein.

Snack: pear – pectin in the pear is good for your gut.

Lunch: pea and mint soup and oatcake and natural yoghurt with sliced banana. Easy to break down fibre and liquid in the soup and probiotic good-to-your-gut yoghurt.

Snack: hummus and carrot sticks – good mix of soluble and insoluble fibre.

Evening meal: chicken with almonds and prunes. Baked apples – rich in pectin which soothes your gut.

Water: aim for about one and a half litres, including peppermint and fennel tea.

Exercise: thirty minutes of exercise, in which you have felt your heart beating faster.

Bonuses: as well as hopefully 'joyous' bowel movements, you will have more energy, a boosted immune system from all the probiotic yoghurt, so no colds or coughs and fantastically clear skin as the extra fibre will remove toxins from the body.

Good Mood Food 8

Just the word 'depression' sounds depressing and I can feel my heart sinking as I write it, so I would rather talk about what puts you in a good mood, makes you laugh, feel good to be alive, think positive thoughts, sleep well, have a good appetite, feel loved and be able to love.

Depression affects about three million in the UK and many of my clients come to see me for depression-associated complaints such as tiredness, overweight, constant colds and trouble sleeping. The exciting thing about the Good Mood Food diet is that it can help all their complaints, including depression, which clients only mention in passing, as if it is something that can only be treated by pills.

Depression is classed as a variety of symptoms: daily mood swings, hyperactivity, crying spells, feelings of despair and hopelessness, loss of pleasure in life, learning difficulties, lethargy, inability to make decisions, insomnia, guilt, anxiety, panic attacks and appetite changes. Depression can also manifest itself as physical aches and pains and digestive upsets. It is perfectly natural to experience some of these symptoms at some time in your life, especially after a traumatic event, so don't read the list and think: 'I was a bit tired yesterday, I couldn't decide whether to wear my Crocs or clogs today, binged on a chocolate chip muffin and got annoyed with Trudy at work, so I must be depressed.'

All around us there is a pressure to be happy – from magazines and television programmes portraying people with perfect lifestyles; satisfying jobs, beautiful homes, lots of friends, compliant relatives and smiling well-behaved children and, if not, stories about those who didn't have those things, but now have. But you can't be happy all the time, you need a bit of 'down' to appreciate the 'up'. You should be allowed to revel in a bit of grumpiness and discontent to then appreciate the good times.

There are, however, serious psychiatric conditions where diet will undoubtedly help, but they might also require medical care and attention so see your doctor if you feel you can't shake off the black cloak of despair. If you are taking anti-depressants, some foods interact, so again that is something you need to discuss with your doctor or nutritionist.

Food is an incredible powerful emotional and physical tool. You can harness it to get the most out of life, winning back control and getting your hormones, neurons and biochemistry on your side – in short, eating yourself back on to an even keel.

Your Brain

Your brain is the control centre of your whole body, influencing all your physical actions from heart rate and breathing to more emotional experiences such as mood and desire. All the time your brain is receiving information, organising and sending messages and storing memories. So it's no wonder your brain gets top priority for oxygen and glucose. Although it only weighs about 1.5kg, it gets one fifth of all your body's oxygen and blood. Your brain is going through myriad physical and emotional actions all the time. Two examples: first, you are cycling along a busy road, not only does your brain control leg and arm movement and balance, but it is also anticipating the speed of the traffic and potential hazards of car doors and stray pedestrians. Second, it can trigger recognition and supply a brief CV of your friend's name and background, coordinate conversation, while at the same time thinking that blue colour doesn't suit them. You may also be thinking 'what will I buy and cook for supper tonight – and what did that woman say in that cookbook that promised I'd feel well?'

All these processes are instigated through an incredible system of electrical impulses. Your brain and spinal cord which constitute your central nervous system are made up of billions of individual nerve cells called neurons. Signals are transmitted through the length of a neuron as an electrical impulse. When a nerve impulse reaches the end of the neuron it has to jump over to the next neuron using chemical messengers called neurotransmitters. Once the message has been conveyed, neurotransmitters are either reabsorbed or destroyed.

When these electrical impulses can't jump efficiently from neuron to neuron your mood and behaviour can change. The major cause of mood swings and depressive symptoms can be attributed to:

- Neurotransmitter imbalance
- Nutrient deficiencies

- Blood sugar imbalance
- Allergies

Neurotransmitter Imbalance

Neurotransmitters are the messengers which carry information between the neurons in your brain. They are made from
amino acids which are made from protein in your food – fish,
meat, pulses, dairy, pulses and grains, so you can see how the
food connection starts and why protein is so important. Your
body can make some of the amino acids, but eight of them are
called essential amino acids as your body has to get them from
food. Here are four of the main mood neurotransmitters which
depend on eating the foods with the relevant amino acids and
vitamins to help conversion.

Acetylcholine = Memory of an elephant Acetylcholine is
involved in memory and mental performance. It keeps your
brain cells supple so that information can pass freely. If levels
fall you can suffer from 'it was on the tip of my tongue' to
complete failure to remember. Acetylcholine is converted from
choline which is found in eggs, cauliflower, lentils, soya
products such as tofu and soya beans and calf's liver. Choline
is also needed to make and maintain the myelin sheath which
is the fat-based protector round nerve cells and ensures fast
and accurate transmission of information. Choline is also
involved in maintaining good gut health.

Dopamine = Get up and Go Dopamine is made from the
non-essential amino acid tyrosine and tyrosine is made from
essential amino acid phenylalanine. Tyrosine can also be
converted to adrenalin and noradrenalin, and along with
dopamine can regulate mood and stimulate metabolism and

the nervous system. Tyrosine acts as an adaptogen which means it can help your body adapt and cope with physical or psychological stress by minimising the symptoms brought on by stress. Good sources are found in soy products, chicken, turkey, fish, peanuts, almonds, avocados, bananas, milk, yoghurt, cottage cheese and ricotta. For the conversion to be effective from phenylalanine to tyrosine to dopamine, or adrenalin and noradrenalin, your body needs folic acid, B12 and magnesium.

GABA = Don't Panic Gamma-Amino Butyric Acid (GABA) has a calming influence, promoting tranquillity and peace. GABA works by steadying the transmission of nerve impulses from one neuron to another. Low GABA levels could mean nerve cells fire too often and too easily. Anxiety disorders such as panic attacks, seizure disorders, and numerous other conditions including addiction, headaches, Parkinson's syndrome, and cognitive impairment are all related to low GABA activity. GABA is found in several food sources, with the highest concentrations being in fish, especially mackerel.

Serotonin = All Is Well with the World Serotonin is made from the essential feel-good amino acid tryptophan. Tryptophan is a large amino acid and it has to compete with other amino acids to make it through the blood/brain barrier – the brain's equivalent of a computer firewall – whose purpose is to separate blood in your body from blood in the brain to prevent substances other than glucose and selected nutrients that could harm the brain getting through. (It's not completely effective as alcohol and caffeine can sneak across). Sweet food encourages tryptophan over the blood/brain barrier, which is why if you are feeling down, your body makes you crave sweet sugary foods to help tryptophan over the barrier.

A better way to access tryptophan is to eat a complex carbohydrate-rich meal. This will trigger the release of the hormone insulin at a controlled rate rather than a surge and once in the brain tryptophan can be converted into serotonin.

The high serotonin levels, in turn, increase feelings of calmness, even drowsiness, regular sleep patterns, increased pain tolerance, and even reduce cravings for carbohydrate-rich foods. People with low serotonin levels can experience insomnia, depression, food cravings, increased sensitivity to pain, aggressive behaviour, and poor body-temperature regulation. Tryptophan is found in eggs, turkey, chicken, bananas, dairy and dates. It also needs vitamin B6 also found in bananas, chicken and wheat germ and complex carbo-hydrates to help process it to serotonin.

Anti-depressants like Prozac are called Selective Serotonin Re-uptake Inhibitors (SSRI) and work on the principle of keeping serotonin circulating in the brain, so they inhibit the re-uptake, allowing the feeling of well being to continue. But they can often have unpleasant side effects. The Good Mood Food way is a natural way to encourage your body to make its own serotonin from tryptophan.

It's All a Question of Balance

Serotonin acts as a counter-balance to tyrosine-induced dopamine and noradrenalin. Serotonin will decrease tend-encies of over-excitement, tension, anxiety and aggression which tyrosine and its derivatives, especially the adrenalins, could produce. Tryptophan and tyrosine create a delicate balance in the brain; a balance that keeps you on a calm and even emotional keel. Often tryptophan and tyrosine occur in the same foods naturally, such as dairy and eggs, so by eating a balanced diet of proteins with complex carbohydrates with enough vitamins to get conversions activated, you can create the balance naturally, so don't get anxious about trying to get the right levels.

Other Ways to Boost Serotonin:

Let There Be Light

The neurotransmitter serotonin and the sleep inducing-hormone melatonin work in partnership. If you don't have enough serotonin and too much melatonin in your body, then you could feel lethargic, find it hard to concentrate and have general low spirits. This is sometimes classed as Seasonal Affective Disorder (SAD). Serotonin levels vary with the seasons and are at their lowest in winter. Melatonin levels go up in the winter which could explain why you feel you have less energy and also a craving for carbohydrates. Serotonin also influences impulse control – so if your levels are low, it's all the harder to say 'no' to a sneaky second biscuit or glass of wine.

Light stimulates serotonin so it is important especially in winter to keep up serotonin levels to avoid feeling sad and lethargic. So as well as eating tryptophan-rich foods and carbohydrates, make sure you get outside for a daily dose of natural daylight. Lux is the measure used for light – on a sunny day you can enjoy 20,000 lux but on an overcast day it can drop down to 7,000 lux and in winter you might be lucky to get 100 lux. If you feel like you just can't get enough light to lift your mood, then it might be worth trying a light therapy box.

> Make sure you get outside for a daily dose of natural daylight

I work in a north-facing, basement office, and we are starved of light, especially in the winter. Then we bought a light box – a flat rectangular box about 600 x 400mm – which emits a steady light of 10,000 lux. We really noticed the difference when it was switched on and so did the coffee and muffin shop across the road – sales must have dropped! You only need to have a light box on for thirty minutes a day. Morning is best, as you need higher melatonin levels at night to induce sleep.

Put on that Tracksuit

Exercise also increases the release of serotonin, so it is good to do something each day that raises your heart rate, especially in the morning. Physical exercise will also help improve the way you cope with stress.

Nutrient Deficiencies

Your brain needs vitamins and minerals to carry out all these amino acid to neurotransmitter conversions.

Vitamin Bs are especially good for the brain. B vitamins don't work independently, so try to make sure you get a good representation. You need to eat the whole range, but it is interesting to see what each one does and how you can access it.

- B1 (thiamine) improves concentration; eat brown rice, wheat germ and soya beans, sunflower seeds.
- B3 (niacin) helps reduce levels of depression and psychosis; eat fish, eggs, wholegrains and poultry.

- B5 (pantothenic acid) improves memory and helps beat stress; eat liver, mushrooms, avocados, egg yolks and wholegrains.
- B6 (pyridoxine) is calming, helps memory and alleviates depression; eat wholegrains such as millet, bananas, buckwheat, oats, chicken, prawns and mussels.
- B12 (cobalamine) prevents confusion; eat meat, fish, dairy and eggs.
- Folic acid guards against anxiety and depression; eat liver, wheat germ, spinach and broccoli and peanuts.

Also:

- Magnesium can be calming and help sleep and is necessary in the production of dopamine; eat sunflower seeds, nuts, green leafy vegetables, soya beans, mackerel and cod.
- Zinc is often implicated in depression especially in post-natal depression as the baby has taken zinc from its mother. Eat oysters, wheat germ, pumpkin seeds and brazil nuts.
- B3, B6 and zinc are the key minerals in depression. B vitamins are all required for memory maintenance, without a good supply of which you could suffer from memory loss, poor concentration and general forgetfulness. They are essential for the cells' energy, especially in the brain.

Fats

Your brain is sixty per cent fat. This fat is in the form of phospholipids which form a layer to protect the neurons – they can act like the insulation on an electrical wire and make sure messages are transmitted smoothly and easily from neuron to neuron. If you eat too much saturated fat or trans fats, then your neurons tend to form clumps in your brain and make neurotransmitters sluggish and sticky or even rigid, whereas if your diet has more unsaturated fats, then the neurons and neurotransmitters can move freely and your brain messaging system flourishes. EPA, found in oily fish, is best for all-round optimum messaging – see Chapter Six, Foods That Hurt – and Those That Heal for more information about EPA. One possible reason for depression is the phospholipid layer in your brain has become thin and is of poor quality, so messages are not as quick and take longer.

In Dr Basant Puri and Hilary Boyd's book *The Natural Way to Beat Depression* (*through EPA*) the authors say it should only take a few weeks to improve the phospholipid layer in your brain by eating more oily fish and foods rich in omega 3 and omega 6 fatty acids, and by cutting right back on saturated fats. Neurotransmitters can then send more messages and at greater speed across the neurons and you should feel – and think – the difference.

Blood Sugar Balance

Your brain consumes more glucose than any other organ. Carbohydrates are broken down to glucose which provides your brain with energy, but you need to eat complex carbohydrates, so that your brain gets an even, steady supply of glucose as sudden fluctuations of glucose can cause mental confusion, dizziness, clouded vision, irritability and headaches. Following the Low Glycemic diet is a good way to guarantee your brain does not suffer from lack of glucose or glucose surges – see Book Tools for more details on managing blood sugar balance.

Carbohydrates are key to helping your body get tryptophan

from food across the blood barrier to your brain to make feel-good serotonin. High-glycemic-index foods can cause blood-sugar swings which will make both your body and your mind irritable and sluggish. Proteins such as oily and white fish, lean meat such as chicken, turkey, pulses and grains combined with carbohydrates help balance your blood sugar as well as providing vital amino acids, so make sure each meal has some carbohydrate and protein with good fats for smooth neuron transmissions.

Allergies

Poor old wheat is always first in the line-up of suspects and the reason why it crops up in the Good Mood Food chapter is that the gluten proteins in wheat mimic endorphins. (Endorphins are natural substances that modify nerve cells and their release is usually stimulated by exercise). The gluten proteins can react with the brain's endorphin receptors in a stimulatory or suppressive way. This can lead to depression, nervousness, loss of motivation and anger. Milk proteins can also react in the same way. Keep a food diary about everything you eat and drink every day, and record your feelings; often it is enough just to cut back and not have wheat or dairy at every meal as both have good vitamins and minerals which can help with your mood balancing.

Good Mood Dos

- Eat foods rich in tyrosine and tryptophan.
- Complex carbohydrates help the uptake of tryptophan and slow down the rate of glucose to the bloodstream.
- Eat oily fish such as mackerel, salmon, herring, sardines and

trout twice a week to get good levels of EPA.

- Take omega 3s (linseed, sunflower, pumpkin and sesame seeds) and omega 6s (lean meat, dairy and sunflower, wheat germ oil).

- Exercise to get oxygen round body, nurturing cells and boosting serotonin.

- Water makes up about eighty per cent of blood and acts as a transport system delivering nutrients to your brain. A common cause of headaches is lack of water. A good guide is to keep topping up water levels all day, so urine is always a pale yellow. Increase liquids if it's hot or if you have been doing exercise, but also make sure you don't lose salts through sweating. Fruit and vegetables, in fact most fresh foods, contain some water and herbal teas count.

- Keep your mind active; socialise and do puzzles – the pub quiz counts, just don't have too much alcohol which will slow down neuron transmission and thought processes.

Good Mood Don'ts

- Avoid foods rich in saturated fats which interfere with blood flow to your brain, so blood cells tend to stick together, making you feel sluggish and slow. Saturated fats can make the cell membrane rigid and brain messaging faulty.

- Reduce refined sugar in your diet as it will play havoc with your brain's blood sugar levels.

- Junk foods and processed food are lacking in vitamins and minerals, and thus eating them will not add to your body's requirement for them, or improve your brain functions. They may even cause your body to use up extra vitamins and minerals to break down the excess sugar.

- Caffeine can increase anxiety and interfere with sleep, so reduce or avoid, but don't stop taking suddenly as you will experience withdrawal effects.
- Alcohol blocks conversion of EFAs and prevents them getting to the phospholipid layer in the brain. Alcohol also causes a sugar rush, so you can feel 'down' an hour later, and then need to keep topping up. Alcohol can increase anxiety levels.
- Smoking impedes the circulation of oxygen to the brain and also destroys vital vitamins for brain health such as Vitamin C and zinc.
- If your adrenal glands get worn out making cortisol and adrenalin, then you are prone to suffer from depression and low motivation. Learn how to deal with stress as it is not always possible to avoid it – see Chapter Four.

Recipes

Cooking is therapy in itself – take your frustration out on chopping a carrot or beating some eggs. Cooking for friends and family, by diverting your mind towards planning and preparation, and through chatting and laughter, will naturally lift your mood.

Spinach and Ricotta Cheese Omelette

This is a lovely light easy breakfast. It is rich in folic acid from the spinach and tyrosine from the eggs and ricotta. In fact, this is ideal to start the day, with all its get-up-and-go tyrosine. This recipe makes enough for two, and is also nice cold, so you could use it as a lunch-on-the-run the following day.

Serves 2

Ingredients

1 tablespoon olive oil

1 small onion, finely chopped

250g frozen chopped spinach

freshly grated nutmeg, to taste

3 eggs, separated

125g ricotta

knob of butter

2 tablespoons freshly grated Parmesan

Method

Heat the olive oil in a large frying pan and cook the onion till soft. Add the spinach and grate in some nutmeg then cover and cook till the spinach is warmed through and wilted. Remove from the heat.

Beat the egg yolks with the ricotta then mix into the spinach and onion.

In a large bowl, beat the egg whites till they form stiff peaks then fold gently into the egg/spinach mix.

Return the frying pan to the heat with a knob of butter. When the butter starts to foam, add the egg/spinach mix and cook gently till just firm to the touch but still moist in the centre – you don't want it too dry.

Preheat the grill to hot, sprinkle grated Parmesan over the top of the omelette and slide it, in the frying pan, under the grill till the cheese turns crispy and golden.

Dr Banana Feelgood Muffins

These double as an excellent snack to sustain you throughout the day and as a speedy breakfast-on-the-move. The banana is a good source of tryptophan and the good complex wholewheat flour and oatmeal mean you don't get a sugar rush – they also help tryptophan across the blood-brain barrier.

Wheat germ, included in this recipe, is the vitamin-rich embryo of the wheat grain and is rich in folic acid and vitamin E; wheat bran is the grain's outer husk. The muffins contain lots of vitamin B, too, in the flour and seeds.

It's a long list of ingredients but all the seeds are worth buying as you will use them in so many other recipes, from muesli, soups and salads to cakes.

Makes 12 muffins

Ingredients

2 ripe, 'spotty' bananas (the riper the banana, the better the flavour)

125g soft brown sugar (weigh out 75g and 50g separately)

150g unsalted butter, softened

3 eggs, beaten

2 tablespoons pumpkin seeds (plus enough to sprinkle on top)

2 tablespoons sunflower seeds (plus enough to sprinkle on top)

1 tablespoon sesame seeds

200g plain wholemeal flour

3 teaspoons baking powder

1 tablespoon wheat germ

2 tablespoons fine oatmeal

1 teaspoon sea salt

Method

Preheat the oven to 180°C/350°F/Gas 4. Grease a 12-hole muffin tin or line with paper cases.

In a medium bowl, roughly mash the bananas with 75g sugar.

In a large mixing bowl, beat the butter with 50g sugar until pale. Gradually add the eggs, beating between each addition. Next, beat in the banana and seeds.

Into a separate bowl sift the flour and baking powder then lightly mix in the baking powder, wheat germ and oatmeal.

Now lightly fold the dry ingredient mix into the creamed butter mix and add the salt. Don't overwork it: the mix should be quite thick and lumpy but happy to drop off a spoon – if you find it's too thick add a little milk.

Spoon into the muffin cases or straight into the muffin tin, sprinkle pumpkin and sunflower seeds atop each muffin and bake in the centre of the oven for 15–20 minutes or till well risen and just firm. Transfer to a wire rack to cool.

Remember, Remember the Cauliflower and Sweet Potato Curry

Cauliflower is a great source of choline, a nutrient thought to contribute to boosting memory. The sweet potatoes here don't just lend their gorgeous colour, they also provide a good source of slow-release energy.

Serve this pretty, orange and creamy white curry with vitamin B-rich brown rice.

Serves 2

Ingredients

2 tablespoons vegetable oil   ½ teaspoon turmeric
1 teaspoon black mustard seeds   2 teaspoons ground coriander

2 teaspoons cumin seeds

1 onion, chopped

knob of ginger, peeled and
chopped

1 sweet potato, scrubbed and
cut in bite-sized chunks

4 tomatoes, skinned and
roughly chopped

1 large cauliflower, divided in
florets

1 teaspoon granulated sugar

100ml hot water

30g slivered almonds, toasted

Method

Heat the oil in a large, shallow, lidded frying pan. When the oil is hot, add the mustard and cumin seeds, put the lid on and wait till you hear the seeds popping – a couple of seconds.

As soon as the seeds have popped, take off the lid, turn down the heat and add the onion, ginger and potato. Cook with lid off till the mixture has softened then add the remaining ingredients up to and including the water. Simmer with the lid on for about 20 minutes till the vegetables are cooked.

Serve scattered with toasted almonds to give a tasty crunch.

Oily fish

Oily fish is the best source of EPA and will do wonders in speeding up nerve transmissions and maintaining a healthy phospholipid layer. Oily fish also provides the nutrients which support healthy vision, learning ability, coordination and balanced moods. EPA can help with weight management and inflammation as well as boost your immune system and balance your hormones.

Memory-Boosting Poached Fish in Lime and Ginger Sauce

While I was working on this chapter of the book I was asked to review some stand-up comedy at the Edinburgh Fringe Festival. I was delighted, till it struck me that I daren't risk writing notes during shows for fear of the comedian mercilessly picking on me. I decided to rely on memory. So for my pre-show supper I made this poached fish dish to sharpen up my brain cells.

The benefit we derive from food is often as much psychological as it is physical: I knew I had done something to improve my memory, therefore I felt confident it would not fail me. As an added bonus all the protein, essential fats and complex carbohydrates in this dish gave me the required stamina for a night out at the Fringe.

This is a lovely, simple way to cook oily fish and enjoy the contrasting flavours and textures of mackerel and salmon plus, of course, all their brain-boosting eicosapentaenoic acid (EPA).

This dish can also be eaten cold.

Serves 2

Ingredients

5 green spring onions, chopped
large knob of fresh ginger,
   peeled and chopped
3 tablespoons fish sauce
4 tablespoons soft brown sugar

juice of 1 lime
500ml cold water
125g salmon fillet
125g mackerel fillet

Method

Put all the ingredients, except the fish, in a large, shallow pan and bring slowly to a gentle simmer. Then add fish and poach till just cooked (about 7 minutes). Lift out the fish using a slotted spoon, cover with foil and keep warm. Bring the poaching broth to the boil and reduce to a dark syrup, then strain.

Serve the fish with the strained syrup spooned over.

Trout Stuffed with Spiced Dates and Barley

Here, you have oily fish rich in eicosapentaenoic acid (EPA), loads of B vitamins in the barley, tryptophan in the dates and some tyrosine in the almonds.

I make the filling in a food processor – the finer it is, the more you can stuff into the trout. If you want to mash up the filling by hand you'll need to finely chop all the ingredients before mixing them.

Serve with green beans.

Serves 4

Ingredients

100g pearl barley
4 whole trout weighing about 500g each, gutted
1 onion, roughly chopped
140g fresh dates

knob of fresh ginger, peeled and roughly chopped
1 teaspoon ground ginger
1 teaspoon ground cinnamon
50g whole almonds, chopped

20g fresh coriander leaves,
  chopped

25g unsalted butter, plus a
  little extra to dot on the fish

Method

Preheat the oven to 180°C/350°F/Gas 4. In a large roasting tin arrange a double layer of lightly oiled foil large enough to loosely parcel up the trout in.

Simmer the pearl barley in water till it is cooked but still has bite to it – about 20 minutes.

Rinse the trout under cold running water and pat dry inside and out. Lay the trout diagonally across the foil in the roasting tin.

In a food processor, blitz the onion then add the remaining ingredients and pulse – don't turn it all to mush, keep it just fine enough to stuff. Fill the gutted cavity of the trout with stuffing and top with a tiny piece of butter.

Close the foil over the trout to make a loose parcel and bake for 20 minutes.

Soya and Serotonin

Soya is a plant oestrogen, and oestrogen plays a huge part in women's mood fluctuations. Levels of oestrogen are associated with low levels of serotonin. A natural way to balance your oestrogen and progesterone levels is to eat foods which have natural plant oestrogen. Soy, tofu, soy sauce, soya beans and soy milk are some of the best examples. Progesterone depresses the activity of the nervous system which in turn prompts an imbalance of brain hormones that influence feelings of depression. This would explain why women feel out of sorts before their periods and during the menopause as progesterone levels are higher and oestrogen lower. Low testosterone has the same effect on men – so boys should eat lots of zinc-rich foods: oysters, red meat, poultry, beans, dairy, nuts and grains and avoid too many soy products if they are feeling low.

Pass Round the Roasted Garlic and Soya Beans

Soya beans are the only vegetable with all eight essential amino acids so they provide valuable brain-building protein as well as some fatty acids, magnesium, folic acid and vitamin B1 plus fibre. You'll find them in the frozen vegetable section of most supermarkets.

This is a great pre-dinner drinks nibble and it takes no more than a minute to prepare. I don't bother peeling the garlic cloves as I like to squish them out over the roasted beans – their lovely rich, soft, sweet intensity perfectly complements the crunchy beans.

Makes pre-dinner nibbles for 4

Ingredients

250g frozen soya beans
olive oil, to coat beans

unpeeled, whole garlic cloves, as many as you like

Method

Preheat the oven to 180°C/350°F/Gas 4.

Toss the beans straight from the freezer onto a baking tray, add enough olive oil to just coat, plus the garlic cloves and roast for 15 minutes till the beans have lost their bright green colour and are crispy but not brown. Lay out on kitchen paper to soak up the oil.

Extract the garlic and squish the cloves with a fork, mix the garlic through the beans and transfer to a bowl.

Buckwheat Noodles with Tofu

No relation to wheat, buckwheat is rich in rutin which has capillary-strengthening properties as well as being a good source of calming vitamin B6. It has a lovely earthy taste which combines well with the fresh tang of the garlic, ginger and chilli-flavoured vegetables and tofu.

Serves 2

Ingredients

150g buckwheat noodles
1 tablespoon vegetable oil
2 spring onions, chopped
knob of ginger, peeled and
    chopped
1 red chilli, deseeded and
    chopped
1 clove garlic, chopped
225g mixed vegetables
    (broccoli, carrots,
    cauliflower, green beans,
    mangetout), cut into bite-
    sized pieces

100ml soy sauce
300ml vegetable stock,
    made with non-additive
    cubes such as Kallo
    organic or Marigold
    Swiss Bouillon powder
300g firm tofu, cut in
    cubes
fresh mint and coriander
    leaves to garnish

Method

Plunge the buckwheat noodles into boiling water and cook for about 10 minutes till soft.

Meanwhile, heat the oil in a large frying pan and stir-fry the spring onions, ginger, chilli, garlic and vegetables for about 5 minutes.

Drain the noodles and return them to the pan along with the cooked vegetables, soy sauce, hot stock and tofu. Stir and heat through.

Serve in soup bowls garnished with lots of mint and coriander.

Fast-Food Chicken Happy Meal

This is a brilliantly easy short-cut supper, ideal when you don't even feel like cooking something to improve your mood. Chicken and sesame seeds are sources of feel-good tryptophan and peanuts contain tyrosine.

Serves 4

Ingredients

Peanut Sauce

250ml apple juice
3 tablespoons no-sugar-added smooth or crunchy peanut butter

juice of 1 lemon
2 tablespoons mango chutney
200g frozen green beans

Chicken

2 tablespoons sesame seeds
2 tablespoons polenta

300g skinless chicken breast,
   cut in bite-sized strips
1 tablespoon vegetable oil

Method

First make the sauce. Heat the apple juice, peanut butter, lemon juice and chutney in a pan and bring to the boil, stirring occasionally, and cook for a couple of minutes. Then add the green beans and cook until just tender and the sauce has thickened.

To prepare the chicken, shake up the sesame seeds and polenta in a plastic bag then toss in the chicken strips and shake till coated. Remove the chicken from the bag and shake off any excess flour.

Heat the oil in a large, non-stick frying pan and shallow fry the chicken till golden brown and cooked through.

Warm up the peanut sauce and serve poured over the chicken.

Tandoori Turkey with Citrus Couscous

Turkey is rich in tryptophan which is converted into anti-depressive serotonin. The yoghurt and lime marinade helps 'cook' the turkey, while grilling the meat on skewers further speeds the cooking process.

Serves 4

Ingredients

150ml natural yoghurt

1 tablespoon curry powder

zest and juice of 2 limes plus
   4 lime wedges to garnish

400g turkey breasts, cut in
   cubes

200g couscous

300ml hot chicken stock

2 tablespoons olive oil

sea salt and freshly ground
   black pepper

4 wooden or metal skewers (soak wooden skewers in water for at least 30 minutes to prevent them burning)

Method

In a shallow dish, mix together the yoghurt, curry powder and the zest and juice from one lime. Submerge the turkey cubes in the yoghurt mix and leave to marinate for 15 minutes.

Next, thread the turkey pieces onto the skewers. Preheat the grill till very hot and grill the turkey skewers, turning once till cooked through (about 4 minutes each side). Set aside, covered to keep warm.

Put the couscous in a bowl, pour over the hot stock and set aside for 5 minutes till the stock has been absorbed. Then gently but thoroughly stir into the couscous the zest and juice from the second lime, the olive oil plus salt and pepper to season.

Serve the turkey skewers on a bed of couscous with wedges of lime on the side.

Little Lemon Ricotta Cakes

The beauty of these zingy little vitamin C-packed cakes is that they are made without flour or butter. Ground almonds and ricotta are both good sources of tyrosine. The egg contains tryptophan, so have a cake to round off a carbohydrate-rich meal and help that tryptophan leap the blood-brain barrier.

Makes 12 cakes

Ingredients

100g ground almonds
400g ricotta
125g unrefined caster sugar
juice of 1 lemon plus
  1 teaspoon lemon rind,
  finely grated

3 eggs, beaten
handful of flaked almonds,
  toasted, to decorate
  (optional)

Method

Preheat the oven to 200°C/400°F/Gas 6. Lightly grease a 12-hole muffin tin.

Put the ground almonds in a large bowl with the ricotta and beat to loosen and mix.

Add the sugar, lemon juice and rind and the eggs and beat till well combined.

Spoon the mix into the muffin tin and bake for 20 minutes or till pale golden and just firm to touch.

Remove from the oven, allow to cool slightly in the tin then run a flat knife around the edge of each cake to loosen it before turning out onto a serving plate. Sprinkle over toasted almonds if you wish.

Get-up-and-Go Ricotta Pud

Easy to make and easy to eat, this tyrosine-rich dessert involves no cooking at all.

Serve with berries to add some vitamin C.

Serves 2–3

Ingredients

2 tablespoons pine nuts,
 toasted
1 tablespoon icing sugar
1 teaspoon ground
 cinnamon

250g ricotta
good quality flower honey
 to drizzle

Method

Toast the pine nuts in a dry frying pan.

Sieve the icing sugar and cinnamon together into a bowl then add the ricotta and beat till smooth.

Spoon a small mound of pudding onto individual serving dishes, drizzle with a little honey and sprinkle over a few toasted pine nuts.

Chocolate Cake to Make You Smile

This lovely chocolate-studded cake can double up as a pudding; glam it up with a little raspberry coulis – just whizz up a punnet of raspberries together with a little icing sugar.

There's no flour or added saturated fats here and the dark

chocolate contains phenylethylamine – which is an essential amino acid and precursor to tyrosine which can, in turn, be converted to feel-good dopamine. Happy eating.

Serves 8

Ingredients

200g dark chocolate,
   70% cocoa solids
4 medium eggs
170g caster sugar

250g ground almonds
1 teaspoon vanilla extract
icing sugar, to dust

Method

Preheat the oven to 170°C/325°F/Gas 3. Line the base of an 8cm deep, 18cm round cake tin with baking paper and grease the sides of the tin with butter.

Chop finely or blitz the chocolate in a food processor to small chunks.

Beat the eggs with the sugar with an electric hand whisk till pale and the consistency of soft marshmallow.

Fold in the chocolate, almonds and vanilla extract.

Pour into the prepared cake tin, and bake for about 20 minutes or till just firm to the touch. Leave to cool in the tin on a wire rack, then turn out and dust with icing sugar.

Good Mood Checklist

- Make sure your diet is rich in EFAs from nuts, seeds, their oils and oily fish.
- Keep the blood sugar balance level with fibre, carbohydrate and protein mix.

- Also a good mix of protein and carbs will help with tryptophan and tyrosine uptake.
- Eat vegetables and fruit for fibre and vitamin C.

Have a Nice Good Mood Day!

Breakfast: start with an oat-based breakfast – muesli, granola or porridge – as oats are a good source of tryptophan and magnesium, which is calming, and B vitamins which help all those neuron conversions. Serve with soy milk or semi-skimmed milk. Or opt for the tyrosine-rich spinach and ricotta omelette.

Snack: banana muffin – good source of tryptophan and vitamin Bs for amino acid conversions.

Lunch: tandoori turkey with citrus couscous – light carbohydrate so not too heavy for the middle of the day and a source of good mood tryptophan.

Snack: nuts and seeds for protein and slow-release energy.

Supper: buckwheat and tofu noodles, and a piece of dark chocolate or chocolate cake. Buckwheat is a good source of calming B6 and the dark chocolate lifts your mood.

Drink: at least one and a half litres of water, neat or as herbal teas.

Exercise: take a brisk walk outside to boost serotonin release and to get your lux for the day to encourage increase of serotonin and less melatonin.

See or phone a friend, talk, laugh and enjoy each other's company.

Bonuses: as well as being in a good mood, you'll have lovely shiny hair, strong nails and good skin from the EFAs, enjoy better sleep and lots of energy and good concentration.

Have a Healthy Heart

From the Soapbox

Many of my clients mention they are taking drugs for lowering their blood pressure as a matter of course, and dismiss it as an inevitable part of life, with a 'Now, let's get back to what is really bothering me' – which could be weight loss, constipation or lack of energy. And this is Scotland, the country with the highest death rate from heart disease in the western world. Scotland used to have a great traditional diet: oatmeal, barley, salmon, herring, lots of root vegetables and now what has happened? Fast food, convenience food and saturated fats – in other words the western diet is to blame. People almost think it is inevitable they will suffer from heart disease. The great news is that you can eat yourself towards a better heart. There is also so much you can do in terms of lifestyle and by addressing weight loss, constipation and lack of energy you can prevent you and your family from suffering from chest pains, breathing and circulation problems and even a stroke or heart attack. And it's never too late, as your heart and blood vessels are capable of recovering from damage.

Your Heart

Your heart is a muscle and functions as two coordinated pumps – one sends blood to the lungs to pick up oxygen and the other pumps oxygenated blood and nutrients round the body. Your heart pumps around 10,000 litres of blood round the body every day through a system of arteries, veins and capillaries delivering oxygen and nutrients to all tissues, muscles and cells. Arteries transport the newly oxygenated blood away from the heart, delivering oxygen to all the cells of your body. Without oxygen for even a few vital minutes these cells would die, so it is vitally important your cells receive oxygen. Veins transport the de-oxygenated blood back towards the heart. Your heart is sort of love-heart shaped – because it is made up of four chambers. The two upper chambers receive blood from the body and the lungs. The lower right chamber pumps blood to the lungs for oxygenation and the lower left chamber pumps blood round the body. The left side is more powerful than the right as it has to pump blood that has been oxygenated to the whole body. A sign of an imminent heart problem can be a pain on the left side of the body, as the heart is struggling to pump blood to the rest of the body. The heart has its own blood supply – two coronary arteries – and these arteries get blocked first.

Blood Pressure

Measuring your blood pressure is the easiest way to detect a potential heart disease. Blood pressure is the force of blood pressing against the walls of your blood vessels. Your blood pressure is at its highest when your heart contracts to push the blood out of the heart through your arteries. This is called systolic pressure. After its exertion, your heart rests, so pressure is lower; this is called diastolic. To take an accurate measure of your heart's activity you need to take two readings – one when your heart is contracting and the other when it is relaxing. These two readings are represented with the highest one first – a typical healthy reading would be 140/80. Your blood pressure varies throughout the day – it is often lowest on waking and rises throughout the day; it also rises as you age. Stress causes your heart to beat faster so you have energy for fight or flight and also physical activity increases your blood pressure as your muscles and cells need more oxygen.

You can eat yourself towards a better heart

A continually high reading for both chambers would suggest that there was some damage to the arteries, as your heart has to exert more pressure to push the blood round the body. High blood pressure can also damage your heart, kidneys and eyes. It's worth keeping tabs on your blood pressure as high blood pressure can also indicate kidney, adrenal and thyroid gland problems as well as explain dizziness, headaches, sweating and headaches and even snoring.

Coronary Heart Disease

Arteriosclerosis 'Arterio' means artery and sclerosis means 'hardening' from the Greek, so arteriosclerosis translates as hardening of your arteries. This happens when calcium salts from the blood are deposited in your arteries, making your blood vessels less flexible, or in fact hard.

Atherosclerosis 'Athero' means 'gruel' or 'paste' in Greek, so your arteries have literally become coated with a thick kind of paste. This paste is made up of low-density lipoprotein (LDL) cholesterol, calcium and platelets which attach themselves to make a thick paste – this is known as furring of the arteries. This paste can thicken and break off and form clots which can cause a stroke or heart attack if they block the artery. Platelets' function is to form blood clots to stop bleeding, but in blood vessels they can stick to the artery walls and contribute to potentially dangerous blockages.

Both these conditions make it harder for your heart to send oxygenated blood round your body, so your blood pressure will increase.

Angina This is experienced as a tightness or heaviness in the centre of the chest and happens when your heart does not receive enough oxygenated blood because the coronary arteries have narrowed through build up of unwanted substances. Sufferers will find that exercise or stress usually triggers angina and that the pain stops when they stop exercising.

A Stroke A stroke is caused by a blood clot either in the brain's blood vessels or in the blood vessels that supply the brain.

Heart Attack Myocardial infarction or cardiac arrest (heart attack) happens when one or more coronary arteries become completely blocked either by being furred up by plaque or by a blood clot.

There are some factors which you can't do anything about which might make you predisposed to heart disease:

- Age – as you get older, the chance of heart disease increases through wear and tear on the blood vessels.
- Gender – men are more likely to get heart disease than women as it is thought oestrogen plays a part in protecting women, but after women complete the menopause the risk balances out.
- Hereditary – if you have a family history of heart disease, then you are at a higher risk of having heart disease.

But there are so many lifestyle changes you can make that you can significantly reduce your risk of getting heart disease. The main things to watch are:

- High blood cholesterol and homocysteine
- Smoking
- Stress
- Caffeine
- Salt
- Alcohol
- Blood sugar
- Overweight and diabetes

Cholesterol
Cholesterol is good – you need it – but in correct amounts. Cholesterol is an important constituent of cell membranes

(outer layers), particularly nerve cells, so is found in every cell of your body. It insulates nerve fibres, and is an essential building block for hormones and vitamin D and also enables the body to produce bile salts which are essential for digestion and absorption of fats. Cholesterol is made in the body, mainly in the liver, but it is also obtained from full-fat dairy products, fatty meat and egg yolks.

Cholesterol is carried around the body by proteins. These combinations of cholesterol and proteins are called lipoproteins. There are two main types: bad and good. High levels of 'bad' low-density lipoprotein (LDL) can lead to the formation of fatty plaques which can narrow the arteries; but there is also 'good' high-density lipoprotein (HDL), which is thought to carry cholesterol away from arteries and back to the liver for processing.

LDL only becomes bad cholesterol if there is not enough HDL to take away the extra cholesterol which forms plaques which stick to the artery walls. When you get your cholesterol checked, you need to know the amounts of LDL and HDL in your bloodstream. Elevated levels of LDL cholesterol may lead to atherosclerosis of the heart and plaque in the rest of the body's blood vessels.

A high intake of saturated fat and lack of exercise can increase the amount of cholesterol produced by the body and so the amount in the blood. Cooking fats and spreads such as butter, margarine, fatty meats and meat products, full-fat milk and dairy products, chips, biscuits, cakes and pastries will all cause an increase in cholesterol. It is far more important to watch your saturated fat intake than worry about cholesterol in foods. As well as cutting back on saturated fats, be wary of trans fat found in processed foods and margarines as they can raise LDL cholesterol levels and so increase the risk of heart disease. Some people have high blood cholesterol even with a healthy lifestyle if they suffer from the inherited condition – familial hyperlipidaemia (FH).

Easy ways to reduce saturated fats are to avoid processed foods and grill, steam, bake, roast food rather than fry. Add herbs rather than butter on your potatoes – or experiment with nut butters on toast rather than butter – nut butters are not butter but whizzed up nuts and you can enjoy in moderation the good polyunsaturated fats founds in nuts.

Fats Are Good

Don't think you should cut out all fat from your diet; your body needs fat to help you to absorb fat-soluble vitamins, make energy, act as insulation, control the passage of compounds in and out of cells, build healthy nerve tissue and form powerful hormones, so don't avoid fats but try to eat good fats. Good fats are polyunsaturated essential fatty acids (EFAs) which are found in oily fish, nuts and seeds. For more information about EFAs, saturated and trans fats turn back to Chapter Six on inflammation. EFAs do not affect blood cholesterol levels but may actually protect against heart disease by making your blood less sticky and less likely to form clots. It is thought that these types of fatty acids also seem to protect against abnormal heartbeats.

Homocysteine

Cholesterol has taken the rap for causing heart disease, but of real concern is an amino acid called homocysteine which can raise the risk of heart disease far more than poor old cholesterol. Homocysteine is made by the body from methionine, an essential amino acid. With the help of B vitamins and zinc, methionine gets converted to glutathione. Glutathione is sometimes called the 'master antioxidant'. In addition to its own antioxidant powers, glutathione can help to recycle other antioxidants such as vitamins C and E. But if your body can't convert the homocysteine to glutathione, you not only miss out on the antioxidant benefits of glutathione, but the homocysteine that accumulates causes build up of plaque in the arteries making the blood thicken and stick to the arterial wall. It also oxidises cholesterol, making it more dangerous. Homocysteine also promotes inflammation in the body and can actually damage arteries and nerves. There is a genetic predisposition to elevated homocysteine levels but diet can reduce levels, by cutting back on animal proteins such as meat and dairy. Make sure you have lots of vitamin B-rich whole-grains in your diet and give up smoking. Blood tests can indicate homocysteine levels.

Smoking

Heavy smokers may have low levels of glutathione as certain chemicals in tobacco smoke increase the rate at which the body uses up glutathione. This makes smokers vulnerable to higher levels of homocysteine. Nicotine constricts the blood vessels, making it harder for the heart to pump blood. The smoke includes carbon monoxide which reduces oxygen levels in not just body tissues but also the heart muscle.

Stress

Too much adrenalin and cortisol (stress hormones) cause the arteries to constrict and cause blood pressure to rise – all ready for fight or flight. See Chapter Four on stress management. These stress hormones make your blood stickier and thicker and ultimately damage the lining of your arteries. Stress also affects calcium and magnesium levels in your body which, as well as the side effects of osteoporosis, also affect the heart muscle as calcium is involved in contraction and magnesium in relaxation.

Caffeine

Heavy coffee drinking has been linked with a rise in cholesterol and homocysteine. But it is thought that while caffeine may temporarily increase blood pressure, the real culprits are substances released during roasting the coffee which cause cholesterol levels to soar. Coffee made in a cafetière or an espresso machine is more likely to increase cholesterol levels than instant or filtered coffee.

Salt

Sodium and potassium work together in your body – sodium works with potassium to help maintain the concentration of body fluids at correct levels. It also plays a central role in the transmission of electrical impulses in the nerves, and helps cells to take up nutrients, so you do need some salt in your body. But if you eat too much salt your blood pressure will be forced up as there will be more water required in your blood which means a greater volume of fluid is passing through your heart. This can in turn place an additional strain on your heart and increases the possibility of coronary disease. Also high levels of fluid circulating through your brain means there is more pressure on your brain's blood vessels which ultimately could cause a stroke.

The best way to reduce your salt levels is to cut

> Coffee made in a cafetière or an espresso machine is more likely to increase cholesterol levels

back on processed food as most salt in the western diet comes from processed foods – prepared meals, crisps, sandwiches, soups, hard cheese, stock cubes, meat extracts, soy sauce, olives in brine, even bread. Also watch out for smoked fish and meats. Manufacturers like salt as it adds flavour cheaply and makes food stay moister for longer. Get in the habit of using less salt when you cook so you can wean yourself off it. Use pepper, spices, herbs or lemon juice instead of salt.

The Food Standards Authority (FSA) recommends 5–6g of salt per day for an adult as the recommended amount – that is one flat teaspoon. It is thought that many people are eating double that amount, and are risking higher blood pressure. And you can see why when an average bowl of cornflakes contains 750mg of salt, one piece of medium sliced white bread contains around 500mg of salt. One portion of tinned soup (half a tin) of soup contains around 2,500mg of salt and a packet of crisps could contain around 1,000mg of salt, which is half the allowance for a six-year-old child. The best way to cut out excess salt is to avoid processed foods as much as possible.

Alcohol

Alcohol can be a friend or foe when it comes to heart disease – a little alcohol, red wine especially, one unit per day (125ml wine, ½ pint beer), could help raise the good high density lipoproteins (HDL) or protective cholesterol and reduce the stickiness of the blood, preventing plaque deposits. But any more is harmful as alcohol is a source of empty calories, so can lead to weight gain and will also raise blood pressure and cause the blood to become stickier. Binge drinking can cause abnormal heart rhythms and regular heavy drinking may lead to enlargement of the heart. If you like a glass of red wine, then enjoy, but don't take to drink!

Overweight

Being overweight can increase your blood pressure as your heart has to work all the harder to pump blood round your body. Excess weight also means that HDL and LDL equilibrium is disrupted. Fat doesn't just get deposited in the cells, more scarily it can get deposited where you can't see it – for example in your arteries. Turn to Chapter One on reducing weight – many of the tools to lose weight will have an impact on reducing the risk of heart disease. Being overweight can also make diabetes more likely to develop.

Diabetes

Diabetes seriously increases the risk of developing cardiovascular disease. Even when glucose (blood sugar) levels are under control, diabetes increases the risk of heart disease and stroke so it is so important that diabetics keep their blood sugar levels under control. Heart disease is the major cause of death for diabetics. See the Book Tools chapter for advice on maintaining constant blood sugar – mainly through regular balanced meals of complex carbs, protein, fibre and good fats.

For a Healthy Heart

There is so much in terms of eating and lifestyle you can do to reduce the chance of suffering from heart disease. Anti-oxidants in food help to protect circulating fats from chemical attack, i.e. oxidation, which triggers the furring up process and can damage cell walls.

Vitamin C is an excellent antioxidant, strengthens the walls of the blood vessels, could help prevent varicose veins and works with bioflavonoids in dark berries and cherries and blackcurrants to strengthen the capillaries. Vitamin C is good for all round heart health and has also been shown to lower cholesterol levels by reducing LDL and increasing HDL which also thins the blood. Fill up on fruit such as mangoes, blackcurrants, strawberries, oranges and vegetables such as green peppers, broccoli and watercress.

Vitamin E reduces platelets sticking together in the blood and lowers blood pressure. It also neutralises free-radical damage. It strengthens blood vessels, regulates heartbeat and increases levels of HDL. It works best with selenium – if you are already taking heart medication such as warfarin which prevents clotting, then don't take vitamin E supplements or excessive amounts of vitamin E food. Eat food with high levels of sunflower oil and seeds, nuts, oats, wholegrains, green vegetables and avocados.

Selenium is needed for the production of glutathione the master antioxidant – selenium amounts are dependent on the soil in which food is grown, but liver, wheat germ, brazil nuts, shellfish, wholegrains and pulses contain some selenium.

Zinc is needed to covert methionine to glutathione to avoid homocysteine build-up and to make hydrochloric acid in the stomach. This in turn affects your ability to taste, so you are less likely to add salt. Zinc is found in oysters, rye, buckwheat, almonds and cashews.

Magnesium helps muscles relax, especially the heart muscle. Magnesium-rich foods are fish, oats, lentils, soya beans, nuts, seeds and green leafy vegetables.

Potassium works with sodium to balance the body fluids. It also plays a vital role in the regulation and functioning of the heartbeat. Most diets are too high in sodium and a diet higher in potassium could reduce blood pressure. Sodium and potassium occur together in many foods, and foods in which the potassium ratio is higher are: raisins, avocados, salmon, bananas, cod, cauliflower, chicken and wholewheat bread.

B vitamins B6 works with B12 to prevent build up of homocysteine. But try and eat the whole range of B vitamins which are found in fish, meat, wholegrains, eggs pulses and greens.

Essential Fatty Acids are found in oily fish, nuts and seeds and can actually reduce blood pressure by making your blood less sticky and less likely to form clots. They also help to reduce weight and promote good HDL cholesterol levels.

Fibre helps to lower cholesterol as it binds to bile acids and removes cholesterol from the body as waste. Turn back to Chapter Seven for more fibre info, but good fibre sources are wholegrains, fruits and vegetables with skins on and pulses. Wholegrains are also a good source of vitamin Bs which are important in combating homocysteine build-up.

Exercise works all your muscles, including your heart muscle which increases its capacity and endurance. Your heart has to beat harder so blood flows faster so more oxygen and nutrients get to your cells. Waste such as toxins and excess cholesterol is taken away. Exercise also increases levels of good HDL cholesterol. Too much physical activity too soon could be a shock to the body and your heart, so aim for thirty minutes a day which leaves you feeling warm and slightly breathless.

Recipes

Food is a powerful ally, but be wary if you are taking medication for high blood pressure not to eat too much garlic and vitamin E-rich foods (or take them as supplements) as they work in the same way as the medication by thinning the blood. Heart disease has become the biggest cause of death in the western world over the last century, mainly due to the huge increase in consumption of processed foods and lack of exercise. But cooking for your heart does not mean bland boring food – spices, especially chillies are good for the heart and the Indian curry spice turmeric has cholesterol-lowering properties.

Breakfast

Start the day with an oat- or barley-based breakfast cereal as they are both rich in soluble fibre beta-d-glucan which will lower cholesterol.

Muesli-on-the-Run Soda Bread

If you don't have time to eat a bowl of muesli in the morning, then try this easy-to-make bread which relies on soda and baking powder to give it 'oomph'.

Luxury muesli with lots of bits in it makes for a more interesting bread, but if your muesli is cereal-heavy, throw in a handful of raisins to bump up the fruit factor.

The bread will keep for about two days. It's great as a snack and it makes good toast, too – or bake it when you have time to enjoy it warm from the oven.

Makes one 500g loaf

Ingredients

250g wholemeal flour
150g of your favourite
    oat-based muesli
1 tablespoon baking powder
1 teaspoon bicarbonate
    of soda

1 teaspoon salt
2 tablespoons vegetable oil
250ml semi skimmed milk
pumpkin and sunflower
    seeds to decorate

Method

Preheat the oven to 180°C/350°F/Gas 4.

Mix all the dry ingredients together in a bowl, add the oil and the milk and stir to make a soft dough – add more milk if necessary.

Sprinkle some flour on your worktop and knead the dough, adding more flour if necessary to achieve a smooth dough. Place the dough on a greased baking sheet and push into a circle about 6cm thick.

Sprinkle some pumpkin and sunflower seeds over the top of the dough and bake in the centre of the oven for 20 minutes till a skewer pushed into the centre comes out clean.

Cool on a wire rack – if you can bear to wait – or eat warm cut into slices.

Grapefruit is rich in pectin which has cholesterol-lowering qualities. Pink-coloured grapefruit is rich in lycopene which can battle with free radicals which cause heart disease. Such is the power of grapefruit that it can affect some prescription medicines. If you are taking statins and calcium channel blockers, for example, check with your doctor before you start eating grapefruit.

New-Look Breakfast Grapefruit

Grapefruit can be quite sharp but this spicy syrup mix makes it a very appealing breakfast option.

Serves 1

Ingredients

1 grapefruit
maple syrup to drizzle

pinch of cinnamon
freshly grated nutmeg

Method

Preheat grill to high. Line the grill pan with foil.

Slice the grapefruit in half. Using a sharp knife, ease the segments away from the surrounding pith and place on a foil-lined grill pan. Drizzle with a little maple syrup, sprinkle over with cinnamon and grated nutmeg then grill till the syrup bubbles.

Garlic has the ability to lower blood cholesterol and prevent clots in the blood vessels and it can also make blood less sticky by keeping the platelets mobile and reducing the chances of clots forming. It is also a valuable antioxidant, so try to include a clove a day in your cooking.

Soup Vegetable soups are a great way to enjoy the fibre and cholesterol-lowering properties of vegetables especially celery, beetroot, aubergine, garlic, onions, peppers and root vegetables. Cut back on oil when cooking by putting the lid on the cooking vegetables, so they cook in their own juices. It is more often habit to make soup with a stock cube. If the ingredients are varied and exciting enough, then you have no need to add extra salt to your soup. Vegetables will naturally contain a balance of minerals such as sodium and potassium from the soil.

Sweet Potato and Carrot Soup

This vibrant, thick orange soup is rich in antioxidants, fibre and vitamin C. What more could a heart wish for?

Serves 4

Ingredients

1 tablespoon olive oil
1 large onion, chopped
1 sweet potato, scrubbed

grated zest and juice of
  1 orange (wash the orange
  before zesting it)

and chopped in bite-
sized pieces
600g carrots, chopped

700ml boiling water
curly or flat parsley to garnish

Method

In a large, lidded pot, heat the oil and sweat the onion –
pan lid on – over a low heat till soft and fragrant. Add the
sweet potato and carrots and stir to mix with the onion.
Add a little water if necessary and let the vegetables
sweat for another 5 minutes.

Add 2 tablespoons of grated orange zest into the
veggie mix, pour in boiling water to cover and simmer till
the vegetables are cooked (about 10 minutes).

Transfer to a food processor and whizz till smooth,
return to the pan, add the orange juice and warm through.

Serve with a garnish of parsley.

Chilli peppers contain substances that have been shown to
prevent clot formation and reduce blood cholesterol and
platelet aggregation. Chillies are a good way to add
flavour if you are cutting back on salt. So be generous with
chillies and also bell peppers; if you add too much, you
can always temper the heat with natural yoghurt – not
water.

Spicy Red Pepper and Chilli Soup

This bright-red soup is full of antioxidant peppers and chillies. Feel free to adjust the amount of chilli you add according to the degree of heat you like.

Serves 4

Ingredients

1 tablespoon olive or sunflower oil

1 large onion, sliced

250g potatoes, chopped

500g red peppers, chopped

1 teaspoon paprika

1 small red chilli, de-seeded and chopped or ½ teaspoon chilli powder

750ml hot water

low fat yoghurt

freshly ground black pepper

Method

Heat the oil in a large, lidded saucepan and gently fry the onion till soft. Add the potatoes, peppers, paprika and chilli and simmer, stirring, for 1 minute. Stir in the hot water and bring to the boil. Turn down the heat, cover the pan and simmer, stirring occasionally, till the vegetables are tender (25–30 minutes).

Allow the soup to cool slightly then pour into a food processor and whizz until smooth. Serve with a swirl of yoghurt and a few twists of black pepper.

Love Your Heart Veggie Tagine

While I was writing this chapter I went to supper with some friends. They served up a glorious veggie tagine, cooked in the traditional, ceramic turret-shaped tagine – theirs was a splendid orange stripy one. And I thought, this ticks all the love-your-heart boxes.

All the vegetables in this recipe contain great fibre for getting rid of excess cholesterol and the spices are great for the circulation. I love the sweet, fruity addition of prunes at the end of cooking. Prunes are good for heart health and, as well as being an excellent source of fibre, they contain compounds which inhibit free radical damage to LDL ('bad') cholesterol.

Don't worry if you don't own a tagine, the recipe tastes just as good made in a casserole dish. Serve the tagine with couscous – fantastically quick and easy to make.

Serves 6–8

Ingredients

Spicy Paste

2 onions, chopped
3 garlic cloves
small knob of fresh root
   ginger, peeled
juice of 1 lemon
100ml olive oil

1 tablespoon each of clear
   honey, ground cumin,
   paprika and turmeric
1 teaspoon hot chilli powder
handful of coriander leaves,
   chopped

Veggie Tagine

1 tablespoon olive oil
3 carrots, cut in chunks
2 sweet potatoes, scrubbed
   and cut in chunks

200g juicy prunes, stoned
   and chopped
400g can chickpeas, drained
400ml hot water

1 red onion, cut in chunks

1 butternut squash, peeled
and cut in chunks

1 leek, ends trimmed and
cut in chunks

2 sprigs mint leaves,
finely chopped

Method

Preheat oven to 200°C/400°F/Gas 6.

First make the spicy paste. Put all the ingredients except the turmeric (it could stain your blender) into a blender and whizz to a thick paste.

Next, put the oil and all the vegetables into a large tagine or ovenproof casserole and cook on the hob, stirring from time to time, till lightly browned (about 10 minutes).

Now add the spicy paste, turmeric, prunes and chickpeas to the vegetables. Pour in 400ml hot water, stir, cover the tagine or casserole with a lid and cook in the oven for 40 minutes. Then reduce heat to 180°C/350°F/Gas 4 and cook for 40 minutes more.

Sprinkle with mint to serve.

Cooking with wine

The Waste Awareness Campaign asked me to give a food demo and tips on not wasting food and one of my suggestions was to freeze leftover wine in ice cube trays. Friends mocked me, who has wine left over? You should finish it, so as not to 'waste' it. If you do have any left though, freeze it in empty ice cube trays, remove when frozen and keep in a freezer bag and add to stews or soups if you want to add some extra body.

Peanut Butter and Red Wine Vegan Stew

My brother once shared a flat with a vegan and they served me this really tasty vegan stew when I went to supper. This dish is full of heart-healthy ingredients.

Vegetables and lentils are great for adding fibre and mopping up cholesterol. Red wine, in moderation, can make your blood less 'sticky'. Peanut butter is a good source of carbs and protein and, when it comes to the heart, it can reduce 'bad' LDL cholesterol and maintain 'good' HDL cholesterol.

Make sure to use peanut butter that has no added salt, sugar or oil – you may need to seek it out in a health food shop as even allegedly 'healthy brands' in supermarkets may have some added palm oil or sea salt. Or you can just whizz up roasted unsalted peanuts in a food processor.

Serves 4–6

Ingredients

2 tablespoons vegetable oil
2 teaspoons whole cumin
  seeds
2 onions, chopped
2 cloves garlic, chopped
100g mushrooms, sliced
400g can tomatoes

225g red lentils
3 tablespoons soy sauce
100ml or 6 'ice cubes' red wine
3 tablespoons crunchy
  peanut butter
2 courgettes, sliced on the
  diagonal

Method

In a large pot, heat the oil, add the cumin seeds and onions and cook over a low heat till the onions soften.

Add the garlic and cook for 1 minute more.

Add the mushrooms, tomatoes, lentils, soy sauce and red wine and simmer for about 15 minutes.

Stir in the peanut butter and add the courgettes 5 minutes before serving so that they are still crunchy.

Spicy Baked Tofu

Soy has been proven to lower total cholesterol and also reduce LDL levels in the bloodstream so it is a good source of protein, especially as you should be trying to shift away from too much animal protein which can be high in saturated fat.

Soy sauce does contain salt, but this recipe has no other added salt. Ginger is great for stimulating the circulation.

Serve either hot or cold with Chinese green vegetables, such as bok choy, and some brown rice to soak up the juices.

Serves 2

Ingredients

1 tablespoon soy sauce
1 teaspoon sesame oil
knob of fresh ginger, peeled
   and grated

2 tablespoons cold water
300g firm tofu, cut in 2cm thick
   squares

Method

Preheat the oven to 190°C/375°F/Gas 5.

Mix the soy, sesame oil, ginger and 2 tablespoons of water together and put in small, ovenproof dish with the beancurd. Let it stand for 10 minutes then bake for 20 minutes, turning once.

Caramelised Butternut Squash and Sweet Potato

All these lovely orange antioxidants will help to see off any free radicals trying to damage your artery walls.

Serve with grilled chicken, grilled fish or spicy tofu and with wholegrains such as amaranth or roasted buckwheat for an extra boost for heart health.

Serves 4 as a side dish

Ingredients

2 butternut squash, peeled and chopped into largish pieces

2 red onions, peeled and cut into wedges

1 sweet potato, scrubbed and chopped into bite-sized pieces

4 cloves garlic

2 tablespoons olive oil

16 cardamom pods

1 tablespoon soft brown sugar

juice of 1 orange

Method

Preheat oven to 220°C/425°F/Gas 7.

Bring a large pan of water to the boil, plunge in the squash pieces, boil for 5 minutes and drain.

In a roasting tin, put the onion wedges, the squash, sweet potato and garlic then drizzle with the oil and shake to coat evenly. Roast in the oven for 30 minutes till gooey and cooked through.

Snip the cardamon pods in half with scissors over a plate and collect the seeds, discard the pods. Crush the seeds using a pestle and mortar, then mix with the sugar and orange juice. Spoon over the hot, roasted vegetables, shake the tin, then return to the oven for 15 minutes more.

Happy Heart Grilled Mackerel with Ginger and Garlic

Omega 3-rich mackerel combined with cholesterol-lowering garlic will fill your heart with joy.

Serve this fast, easy-to-cook supper with lime wedges for extra vitamin C and brown rice for vitamin B. There are lots of strong flavours here, so no need to reach for the salt.

Serves 2

Ingredients

2 tablespoons fresh ginger, peeled and finely chopped
2 tablespoons garlic, crushed
2 tablespoons fresh lime juice, plus lime wedges to serve

1 tablespoon vegetable oil
2 mackerel fillets, skin on

Method

Combine the ginger, garlic, lime juice and oil together in a small bowl then rub all over the mackerel flesh and set aside to marinate for at least 10 minutes: the lime juice will 'cook' the fish slightly and you will see the flesh turning white.

Grill mackerel, skin side down, for about 7 minutes till lightly browned. There is no need to turn the fish.

Serve with lime wedges.

Chicken and Almond Barley Pilaf

A great cholesterol-lowering dish thanks to the onions, garlic and carrot plus the barley – a great source of soluble beta-d-glucan – another cholesterol-buster.

Serves 2

Ingredients

1 tablespoon olive oil
2 onions, chopped
1 clove garlic, finely chopped
225g skinless chicken breast,
  chopped into bite-sized pieces
1 large carrot, cut in thin
  matchsticks

50g dried, unsulphured
  apricots, cut in small pieces
280g pot or pearl barley
1 teaspoon cinnamon
3 tablespoons raisins
700ml water
50g flaked almonds, toasted

Method

In a large pot, fry the onions and the garlic in the oil until they begin to brown. Stir-fry in the carrot and apricots.

Add the chicken pieces and sauté till lightly browned and cooked through.

Add the barley, cinnamon, raisins and hot water then

simmer till the barley is cooked – add more water if necessary to prevent the stew catching.

Stir in the toasted almonds just before serving.

Fruit Creamy desserts are not kind for heart watchers as they tend to be high in saturated fat and also calories. I feel I'd rather have a tiny piece of the real thing, than a half-hearted low-fat effort, but fruit is wonderful for the heart. Pectin is a soluble fibre that can lower cholesterol through decreasing both the absorption and synthesis of cholesterol, and is found in apples, bananas, grapefruit, oranges and pears. Two pieces of fruit per day have enough pectin to make a significant impact on reducing heart disease. Try to get in the habit of making fresh seasonal fruit salad for you and your family to end a meal. Chop just before serving and squeeze some orange juice over to help prevent oxidation.

Banana, Date and Hazelnut Oat Crumble

Bananas are a good source of potassium which is vital for heart muscle function.

Dates and oats are a source of soluble fibre and of beta-d-glucan, which may decrease the body's absorption of cholesterol. Nuts and seeds are good for heart health as they are rich in essential fatty acids, plus hazelnuts contain high levels of copper. Copper is a key component of an antioxidant enzyme which can disarm the free radicals which would otherwise damage cholesterol and other lipids. Oats are also rich in magnesium which relaxes nerves and muscles, including the heart muscle, so this is a good pud to have in the evening before going to bed.

Serves 4

Ingredients

Crumble Topping

75g cold, unsalted butter, cut in small chunks

100g soya or wholewheat flour

50g rolled oats

50g hazelnuts, chopped

75g soft brown sugar

1 teaspoon ground ginger

zest of 1 lime

Filling

2 bananas, chopped

100g fresh dates

knob of fresh ginger

25g soft brown sugar

juice of 1 lime

Method

Preheat the oven to 170°C/325°F/Gas 3.

Put all the crumble topping ingredients in a large bowl and make the crumble by rubbing the chunks of butter through your fingers with the dry ingredients till it resembles a crumb-like consistency.

For the fruit base, in a greased ovenproof dish, put the bananas, dates and ginger then mix in the sugar and lime juice.

Spoon the crumble topping over the fruit and bake for about 20 minutes till the crumble topping turns golden brown.

Grapes are very high in flavanoids which can help with reversing atherosclerosis. Grapes also contain a group of compounds called resveratrol which acts like an antioxidant and can reduce the build up of plaque in arteries. They're high in sugar, so eat as part of a meal to avoid disrupting blood sugar balance.

Freeze-Me-A-Grape Serve frozen grapes as a dessert, wash well and pat dry and arrange on a single baking tray and place in the freezer. Once frozen keep the grapes in a freezer bag and serve straight from the freezer. They look very pretty if you freeze red and green grapes and serve them together.

Pears Poached in Red Wine

This is a very pretty and sophisticated dinner party pud – and your kitchen will smell lovely as the spiced wine gives off a wonderful aroma as it simmers. When I first made this dish I served it with a slice of creamy Gorgonzola, which was heaven – sorry, I shouldn't have mentioned this, but if you are giving yourself a day off then at least the pears and red wine will help towards balancing the saturated fat and LDL of the cheese. Pears, even peeled, are a good source of cholesterol-lowering pectin. Red wine in small quantities can help to make blood cells less 'sticky' and may encourage 'good' HDL cholesterol.

Serves 6

Ingredients

6 pears, peeled but not
   cored (leave the stalk on)
600ml red wine
225g soft brown sugar
1 teaspoon black peppercorns
pinch grated nutmeg
pinch ground cinnamon
1 teaspoon coriander seeds

1 clove
juice of 1 lemon
juice of 1 orange plus the zest,
   finely grated
2 tablespoons redcurrant jelly
knob of ginger, peeled and
   grated

Method

Put all the ingredients in a large pan and simmer with the lid off for about 30 minutes till the pears soften (you should be able to slide a sharp knife into them easily). Remove the pears with a slotted spoon and stand them in a large, shallow bowl.

Turn up the heat under the spiced wine so that it reduces by about 1/3 to a syrup. Pour the syrup over pears in the bowl and leave to cool. Serve cold with a little of the syrup on each pear.

Healthy Heart Checklist

Include in your diet

- EFAs – lots of oily fish, nuts and seeds and nut and seed oils.
- Green and root vegetables and pulses to maintain an alkaline balance in the body and for adequate fibre to help remove excess cholesterol from the body.
- Fresh fruit as it is high in pectin and vitamin C.

- Avoid junk, processed refined carbohydrate foods which could be high in sugar, salt and saturated fats.
- Cut back on alcohol.
- Cut back on sugar.
- Don't add salt to food.
- Eat less animal protein so less dairy and meat.
- Reduce caffeine to reduce homocysteine.
- Exercise – try for thirty minutes a day.
- Don't smoke.

Have a Healthy Heart Day!

Breakfast: grilled grapefruit and porridge with pumpkin and sunflower seeds and sliced pears and blueberries – start the day with cholesterol-lowering oats and vitamin C and fibre-rich foods.

Snack: rye bread toasted with peanut butter and sliced bananas – filling slow-release energy snack with cholesterol-lowering peanuts and magnesium-calming bananas. Eating bananas with slow-release bread and peanut butter slows down their fast-release sugar.

Lunch: spicy red pepper and chilli soup and an oatcake – cholesterol-lowering spices and fibre.

Snack: guacamole – avocado dip with carrot sticks – potassium-rich snack.

Evening meal: grilled salmon with butternut squash with cardamom and orange and banana, hazelnut and oat crumble. EFA-rich salmon and antioxidant-rich squash followed by relaxing cholesterol-reducing crumble.

Exercise: brisk walk to get your circulation going.

Bonuses: shiny hair, strong nails, good mood from increased EFAs in your diet, good bowel movements due to the extra fibre, and clear toxin-free skin.

Some Things Are Worth Getting Fat For

10

This is like my *Desert Island Discs* of favourite naughty foods – and I have to say most of them involve cream, butter, cheese, sugar and even whisky. And we all know, after reading nine chapters, they will send your blood sugar sky-high, your collagen will crumble at the onslaught of so much glucose, your brain could go into potential meltdown, your joints will inflame and you'll break out in some kind of rash.

But you won't, just don't eat the whole cake/muffin/all the scones and don't do it every day.

A slim, stylish friend who loves food has a question she asks herself when she sees something she is tempted by, usually a sweet: 'Is it worth getting fat for?' It's a very good question, as it makes you stop and think about the piece of gooey chocolate brownie rather than saying 'I'll take two with extra cream ...' Weigh it up in your mind.

- Is it homemade? Look for tell-tale commercial tinfoil packing and suspiciously even sizes.
- Is it fresh? Does it look dried up at the edges? Butter icing can go thin and streaky. Cake can dry out, especially if you get an outer piece.
- Is it really gooey/creamy/fudgey? Fresh whipped cream flops over, fudge topping should be shiny.
- Is it really worth getting fat for?

It helps if you can see the cake in question and nine out of ten times, you'll decide not to have it. You will enjoy an incredible feeling of superiority and control; you have taken on the double dark forces of brownie and won!

But if you really want to sink your teeth into the soft all-enveloping chocolate, you know what it means: there will be calories to burn off, you'll have to go up a notch on the belt and it'll be another week before you'll want to go swimsuit shopping. But if this cake is worth it, the pleasure will outlive the consequences, you will remember the taste, sensation, the flavour for days, weeks, maybe even years to come; so have it – and enjoy – with no guilt. Guilt and remorse are not part of the Some Things Are Worth Getting Fat For Plan.

I've spent hours looking back at all my old recipe books and ransacking my food memory banks and all the recipes here definitely Are Worth Getting Fat For. But they are still made of good wholesome ingredients: butter, cheese and cream. Even though they are full of saturated fat, they are also a good source of calcium, protein, vitamin A, zinc, potassium, omega 6 and energy. Even sugar can give you a sugar burst, when you are flagging, and I've also squeezed in some ingredients which are always good for you such as beetroot, ginger, dates, whole-wheat bread, eggs, strawberries and hazelnuts. And it's not all sweets and puddings either – I've included some indulgent main courses too, ideally not to be eaten all on the same day!

Ingredients

It's all about quality and treating yourself, as this won't happen this often, will it? So buy the best.

Butter Butter has very little going for it nutritionally – but it does have good levels of vitamin A. It is a very saturated fat which can conflict with your good omega 3s and is high in calories, so be sparing with it and see it as a treat. As it is a certified treat, buy the best – I like the European style unsalted butter – which is rich, creamy and intensely satisfying. Butter is made by churning cream until the fats separate from the liquid, leaving a liquid – buttermilk – and a semi-solid mass. This can then be shaped and chilled. Most butter is made from cow's milk but butter can also be produced from the milk of any animal. European style butters have a slight tang from a lactic acid culture that is added to the cream. Salted butter tends to last longer than unsalted, as the salt acts as a preservative – you can sometimes see the outer edge go a darker yellow as it oxidises.

Cheaper butters may be dyed yellow, but the cows' diet will also affect the colour, reflecting the change in seasons. More expensive butter means the cows may have been raised in more humane conditions, fed on better quality food – grass, silage and hay, which will be reflected in the quality of their milk, cream and butter. Be wary of cheaper blended butters and butter from more than one country as the cows may well have been fed on cheaper food and hormones to boost milk production. Reduced fat butters are made by including vegetable oils and sometimes water, but the flavour will be compromised. Have the real thing.

Sugar Sugar consists entirely of carbohydrate – mainly sucrose – and has no fibre, vitamins or minerals. White commercial sugar is a refined sugar derived from sugar cane and sugar beets. It is sold in many granule sizes ranging from icing sugar to granulated. All through *Eat Well with Nell*, brown has been best – rice, flour, pasta – because it is less processed and should contain more vitamins, minerals and fibre. But when it comes to sugar, sadly this mantra does not hold true. There is very little significant nutritional difference between white and brown sugar. Most brown sugar is simply refined white sugar coated in molasses which is added during processing. Unrefined brown sugar has undergone the minimal processing necessary to make sugar from the cane plant and will have some natural molasses. I use brown sugar, especially in cakes, as I like to think I can taste the richer toffee-like flavour of molasses. The darker the sugar, the darker the end product, so it's great for dark gooey-looking brownies. Meringues are traditionally made with white caster sugar, but brown meringues have a lovely homespun look about them and again the more toffee-like flavour.

Manufacturers like sugar as it is a comparatively cheap ingredient; it adds flavour to foods – both sweet and savoury – and sugar's ability to hold moisture means it prolongs the shelf life of baked goods. Bought cakes may well have more sugar in them than homemade, as well as more salt and saturated and trans fats which all act as preservatives ... so if you are going to eat cake, why not make your own?

Butter and Baking You can wean yourself off adding butter to food, but for baking it is necessary. Butter adds flavour and texture to your baking and helps to keep it fresh. The temperature of the butter is very important in baking. Many recipes require butter to be at room temperature as this allows the maximum amount of air to be beaten into your mix. Creaming butter and sugar creates air bubbles that your raising agent will enlarge during baking. Most experts recommend four to five minutes of creaming the butter for maximum aeration. Cold butter is recommended for pastry so less butter is absorbed by the starch in the flour, so you get layers which make your pastry flaky and less dense. It is best not to use butter that has been frozen for baking, as freezing can affect the texture of the butter and change its moisture content. When cooking with butter don't be tempted to use reduced fat butter as some have water added to reduce the fat content and this will affect the dynamics in the oven.

Sugar and baking When sugar is used in baking its role becomes more complex as it also adds volume, tenderness, texture, colour, and acts as a preservative. Brown sugar has slightly different qualities.

When a recipe calls for creaming together the fat and sugar, this is to get air into the mix as the sugar granules rub against the fat producing air bubbles. When you add the raising ingredient, the gases enlarge these air bubbles and cause the mix to rise when put in the oven. The length of time you cream the butter with the sugar determines the amount of air incorporated into the mixture.

Sugar, especially brown sugar, attracts water so it competes with the gluten-forming proteins in the batter which also like liquid so they can form bubbles of air which will make your cake or bread light. Without the 'thirsty' sugar, the gluten could form too many more solid pockets, which could make your cake rigid and less light.

The size of the sugar crystal affects the amount of air that

❝ Don't feel guilty, enjoy and revel in every spoonful **❞**

can be incorporated into the mix during the creaming of the sugar and fat. Granulated sugar will incorporate more air into the mix than icing sugar, so it is best for general baking, whereas caster sugar is basically superfine granulated sugar, good for making meringues as it dissolves rapidly. You can make your own caster sugar by processing granulated sugar in your food processor for a few seconds. Icing sugar is very finely ground granulated sugar with some cornflour added to prevent lumps forming.

Sugar also reacts with the protein in other ingredients such as the eggs and milk when heated to cause a browning effect; the higher the sugar content the darker the crust. Brown sugar has the tendency to lump and become hard. Brown sugar should be stored in a thick plastic bag in a cool, dry place.

Recipes

Indulging

If you are going to indulge yourself, go for the middle ground; enjoy a well-balanced first course then, when you do go in, cake fork flying at the ready, your blood sugar won't rocket. The solid base of carbohydrate, protein and fibre will balance the sugar surges and also prevent you going back for second helpings and so help minimise calorie intake.

Don't feel guilty enjoy and revel in every spoonful, sit down and savour the moment. There is always tomorrow to get back on the straight and narrow – in every sense.

None of these recipes are for one. Remember the maxim

'share the calories' and view food as a real pleasure to share with family and friends.

Oyster, Steak and Ale Pie

This delicious pie owes its origin to the days when oysters were so plentiful that they were added to stews and pies to 'make the meat stretch'. Filming *The Woman Who Ate Scotland* was a wonderful chance to sample so much of the best of Scottish food and for the episode on Argyll we visited Loch Fyne and its splendid oyster bar for a lesson in oyster opening and eating.

The family-run brewery Fyne Ales is just around the corner from the oyster bar so we bought some of their Vital Spark dark ale and I pedalled down to the Kilfinan Hotel to make this traditional pie using local beef. Traditionally porter, which is a very dark ale, would have been used in this pie but any dark ale will do.

If you have a plentiful supply of oysters, or a healthy bank balance, then use freshly opened oysters. Or use a tin of smoked oysters, which is almost as good, cheaper and a lot easier to open! Oysters are incredibly rich in zinc so they'll give your immune system a boost.

Serve with some greens and a creamy potato gratin which you could cook in the oven at the same time.

Serves 4

Ingredients

3–4 tablespoons olive oil

400g stewing steak, cut in bite-sized chunks and tossed in a tablespoon of seasoned flour

a few sprigs of fresh thyme

900ml dark ale

2 cloves garlic, finely chopped

8–12 fresh oysters, shucked or 1 can of smoked oysters

knob of butter

5 shallots, skinned and
   chopped

200g unsmoked bacon,
   roughly chopped

375g ready-to-roll puff pastry

1 egg, lightly beaten

Method

Preheat the oven to 200°C/400°F/Gas 6.

Heat the oil in large, lidded, flameproof casserole dish (or heavy-based pot) and fry the beef (dusted in flour) over a medium heat until browned all over. Remove the beef and set aside.

Melt the butter in the casserole dish and add the shallots, bacon and sprigs of thyme and sauté for about 5 minutes, then stir in the ale. Simmer for 5 minutes then return the beef to the pan, add the garlic and stir to mix through. Cover and cook slowly on the hob for 1 hour 30 minutes. Then add the oysters to the casserole.

Transfer to an ovenproof casserole dish and fill it three-quarters full with beef and oyster mixture.

Roll the puff pastry out to cover the top of the dish and crimp the edges neatly. Brush with beaten egg and bake for 25–30 minutes, till the pastry is risen and golden.

Kaffir Lime and Gorgonzola Risotto

I was editor of the food magazine *Asian Home Gourmet* in Hong Kong at the peak of the craze for fusion food – a not always successful marriage of east meets west: sometimes it was a head-on collision of cultures and other times it was an amazing combination of the best of both hemispheres. This recipe is an example of the best of both. The risotto is based on one that chef Brian Nagao of The Peninsula's Felix Restaurant made for the magazine. I think its success is due to the sheer gorgeousness and limeiness of the Thai kaffir lime leaf which works so brilliantly with the rich creaminess of the Gorgonzola, set against a backdrop of buttery rice. Fresh kaffir lime leaves are essential for this dish and you may need to head to a Thai produce shop, as dried leaves just don't have the same flavour.

Serves 4

Ingredients

knob of butter

120g onions, chopped

4 fresh kaffir lime leaves, plus a couple cut in strips to garnish

500g risotto rice such as arborio or carnaroli

50g butter

1 litre hot chicken stock

150g Gorgonzola, cut in rough chunks

Method

In a deep, heavy-based pan, melt the knob of butter and sauté the onions and kaffir lime leaves together then add the rice and cook for a few minutes till the grains are coated and glossy.

Add the hot chicken stock gradually, one ladle at a time, stirring with each addition till the rice absorbs the stock.

When all the stock has been added and the rice just begins to give in to your bite, stir in the chunks of

Gorgonzola and allow to melt slightly. Stir in the remaining butter.

Serve with a few strips of lime leaf as a garnish.

Slow-Cooked Pork with Wine, Cider and Cream

This is a gorgeous marriage of tender marinated pork, wine-stewed prunes, cream and a burst of colour and zest from the scarlet cranberries.

This recipe is adapted from a dish served at a wonderful restaurant not too far from North Berwick, where I grew up, called La Potinière – which, sadly, is no more. For a person, like me, who suffers from neighbouring-table food envy, La Potinière was extra wonderful: there was a set menu so it was like going to dinner at a friend's house – no menu agonising.

The prunes in this recipe are a great source of fibre and can help reduce LDL ('bad') cholesterol which, you can be sure, is in the cream and the pork so you could call it a 'pay off'. To try and offset some of that cholesterol damage still more, serve with cooked spinach or a sweet potato gratin.

Serves 6

Ingredients

860ml cold water

50g soft brown or demerara sugar

50g sea salt

6 double loin pork chops, fat trimmed off

knob of unsalted butter

350ml dry cider

250g plump prunes

300ml dry white wine

225ml double cream

50g frozen cranberries

Method

Heat the water with the sugar and salt till both have dissolved. Bring to the boil and boil for a few minutes then pour the water into a bowl large enough to take it and the chops. Let the water cool and when cold, submerge the chops and leave overnight in the fridge.

Preheat the oven to 150°C/300°F/Gas 2.

Remove the chops from the bowl and pat dry with kitchen towel. Melt the butter in a large frying pan and when hot, but not burnt, fry the chops quickly on both sides to seal in flavour. Transfer to an ovenproof dish (with a lid).

Pour the cider into the frying pan, bring to the boil, then pour over the chops. Cover and braise for 3 hours, checking occasionally to make sure the chops don't dry out – if they look as if they are drying out, add some water or some more cider.

Meanwhile, place the prunes a large ovenproof dish, add the white wine, cover to prevent evaporating and cook in the oven at the same time as the chops for an hour.

When cooking time is up, remove the dishes of prunes and chops from the oven. Pour the chops' cooking liquid into a jug and let it sit for about 10 minutes till the fat rises.

Blot off the fat off the chop liquid with kitchen towel then pour into a pan on the hob, along with any prune and wine liquor – don't waste any! Bring to the boil and let it reduce a little. Add the cream and allow to simmer very gently for 5 minutes so you have a gorgeous creamy rich sauce.

Just before serving, add the cranberries to the cream

sauce and allow to heat through – don't let it boil or the berries will burst.

Serve each chop on a warmed plate with the sauce and prunes on the plate.

Sticky Toffee Pudding

This is the ultimate comfort food. The name is brilliant – date sponge, which is what it is, would never instigate, 'Go on, I'll have some date sponge, if you'll have some.' Just that name 'sticky toffee pudding' is a clarion call for most pudding lovers.

You can bake it in a cake tin and serve it in portions, or in a muffin tin to make individual cakes. I've doubled the usual sauce amounts as I love my sticky toffee pudding almost swimming in sauce. And I like it with thick double cream . . . If you're going to do it, do it in style, then hit the green leafy salad and cholesterol-absorbing oats tomorrow.

Serves 6

Ingredients

Sponge

50g unsalted butter
175g caster sugar
2 eggs, beaten
175g dried dates, chopped
300ml boiling water
1 teaspoon bicarbonate of soda
175g self-raising flour
1 teaspoon vanilla extract

Toffee Sauce

150g butter   200g soft brown sugar
100ml double cream

Method

Preheat the oven to 180°C/350°F/Gas 4. Grease a 20cm baking tin or 12-hole muffin tin.

Cream the butter and sugar together in a food processor till pale and creamy, then add the eggs, gradually, whizzing after each addition.

Put the dates in a bowl, pour over the boiling water and stir to break down, then add the bicarbonate of soda and allow to cool slightly. Once cooled, add the dates and water along with the flour and vanilla extract, to the creamed butter and sugar. Stir to mix.

Pour the mixture into the baking tin or muffin tin and bake in the centre of the oven for 20–30 minutes till firm to touch.

To make the toffee sauce, gently heat the butter, double cream and brown sugar in a small thick-based pan. Serve the sauce hot, poured over hot sponge.

Brown Bread Ice Cream

You think I've lost it and all this nutritional business has got to me but I promise you, white bread ice cream would taste horrid. Vile Brown bread ice cream was very popular in Victorian times but I think it is definitely due for a – tasteful – revival. Brown breadcrumbs are toasted with hazelnuts and brown sugar and you get this wonderful caramel mixture that permeates right through the rich double cream.

Serves 4

Ingredients

50g hazelnuts

100g fresh, wholemeal
  breadcrumbs

50g muscovado sugar

4 eggs, separated

100g golden caster sugar

300ml double cream

Method

Whizz the hazelnuts in a food processor till they resemble big breadcrumbs. Lay the nuts, breadcrumbs and muscovado sugar on a baking tray and toast under a hot grill till they have metamorphosed into caramel nuggets.

Whisk the egg yolks in a bowl. In a separate bowl, whisk the egg whites till stiff then gradually whisk the sugar into them.

Then, in another bowl, whisk the cream till it forms soft peaks, then fold it into the egg white mix. Next, fold the egg yolks, and then the caramel nuggets, into the cream and egg white mix.

Pour into a container with a lid and freeze overnight. Remove from the freezer at least 15 minutes before serving to let it soften.

Whisky Mac Cheesecake

On a cold, wet day I love to drink a Whisky Mac – whisky with a shot of green ginger wine. I've celebrated several very happy

Burns Nights and Hogmanays in Hong Kong and Scotland with this Whisky Mac-inspired pud.

The spice of the ginger and the alcohol of the whisky cut through the almost cloying creaminess of the mascarpone in this recipe.

Serves 8

Ingredients

Cheesecake Base

240g ginger biscuits   120g unsalted butter

Whisky Mac Filling

400g full fat cream cheese   6 pieces of stem ginger
250g mascarpone   plus syrup
180g caster sugar   4 tablespoons whisky
4 eggs   (or to taste)

Method

Preheat the oven to 150°C/300°F/Gas 2.

Pulverise the biscuits – the best way is in a food processor, or put them in a tough plastic bag and smash with a rolling pin. Melt the butter, add the biscuits to the butter and mix, then press into a greased, loose bottom 20cm cake tin. I find it too hard to go up the edges, so covering the base is fine.

To make the filling, put all the ingredients up to and including the eggs into a food processor and whizz. Then quickly pulse the pieces of stem ginger. Add in about 2 tablespoons of ginger syrup and 4 tablespoons of whisky, mix through, taste and add more if necessary.

Pour onto the prepared base and bake in the centre of

the oven for 30–40 minutes till just set. You can leave the cheesecake in the oven overnight to cool down gradually.

Good Morning Hot Cheese Scones

After my first few school summer holiday jobs – strawberry picking, newspaper rounds and a very brief stint as a washer upper in an ice cream bar – I finally landed a summer job as a waitress. It was in a small café in North Berwick, a seaside town twenty miles from Edinburgh, where I grew up.

Each morning, one of the local ladies would come in to bake scones and pancakes for the café. It was my favourite time of the day – there were no customers to clutter up the café, ruining cake displays and spilling things. The windows were condensation-clear, the carpet crumb-free, the coffee machine was hyperventilating fresh coffee and from the oven came trays of piping hot cheese, floury plain and fruit-studded scones.

The mustard in this recipe gives the scones a real kick, and it's worth using a good, crumbly, full-flavoured Cheddar cheese.

Makes 9 scones

Ingredients

350g self-raising flour
½ teaspoon sea salt
1 teaspoon baking powder
2 teaspoons dry mustard
   powder

250ml milk, plus extra for glazing
1 egg, beaten
125g strong Cheddar cheese,
   grated
cold, unsalted butter to serve

Method

Preheat the oven to 220°C/425°F/Gas 7.

Make these by hand for the dough-under-the-finger-nails experience, or whizz them up in a food processor – the trick is to handle the dough as little as possible.

Sieve the dry ingredients together into a bowl then add the milk, egg and cheese. Bring the mixture together with your hand and gently knead – it is sticky.

Shape and lay the dough directly onto a floured baking tray and score into 9 squares, or gently press the mixture out on a floured surface till it is about 3 cm thick and stamp out rounds with a cutter, then transfer to the floured baking tray

Brush a little milk over the top of the dough to glaze or sprinkle on a little grated cheese. Bake in the centre of the oven for 10–15 minutes till well risen and golden brown. Serve hot, split in half and spread with butter straight from the fridge.

Strawberry and Cream Cheese Muffins

I first tasted strawberry and cream cheese muffins when a group of us were cycling round the coast of New Zealand's North Island. It was pouring with rain when we finally got to a small town called Coramandel. When we took shelter in a café there, these muffins were being brought out the oven – sweet, warm nuggets of strawberries nestling in pockets of molten cream cheese within ethereally light sponge. I remember the absolute joy I felt when I tucked into these muffins and drank a steaming caffe latte by a roaring hot fire.

Makes 6 huge muffins

Ingredients

300g self-raising flour
125g caster sugar
¼ teaspoon salt
125g butter, melted
125ml cold water

1 egg, beaten
275g strawberries, hulled and finely
  chopped
250g cream cheese, cut in little cubes

Method

Preheat the oven to 200°C/400°F/Gas 6. Grease only the base of the muffin tin, not the sides, otherwise the muffin mixture won't be able to get a grip to rise.

Sieve all the dry ingredients together. Melt the butter then, in a large bowl, mix together with the water and egg.

Very gently, and using a fork, fold the dry ingredients into the egg and water, taking care not to overmix. Add the chopped strawberries and cubed cheese, mix and spoon into the muffin tin, filling almost to the top.

Bake for 15–20 minutes till golden brown and risen. Cool for 5 minutes in the tin, then remove to a wire rack.

Millionaire Toffee Shortbread

When I was cycling from Hong Kong to Sydney, all it took was one bite of toffee shortbread in a caravan park in New South Wales, Australia to decide I was 'dun roamin''. I was heading back to Scotland – the land of toffee shortbread.

Eat this in small quantities and, ideally, at the end of a meal to help ease the huge sugar burden.

Shortbread

125g butter   175g plain flour
75g sugar

Caramel

395g can condensed milk   100g butter
2 tablespoons golden syrup

Topping

85g dark chocolate, 70% cocoa solids

Method

Preheat the oven to 180°C/350°F/Gas 4. Grease a 4cm deep, 20cm square baking tray.

Cream the butter and sugar together then mix in the flour to form a ball. Press into the baking tray and bake for 12–15 minutes, till pale golden. Leave to cool in the tray for 10 minutes.

Meanwhile, make the caramel. Put all the ingredients in a heavy pan and bring slowly to the boil, stirring all the time. Boil for 3–7 minutes, stirring occasionally, so it does not stick, until it has darkened to a glorious golden caramel, but not coffee fudge colour. Remove from the heat, place pan on a cloth soaked in cold water and stir briskly for 2–3 minutes. Spread over the shortbread and allow to cool.

To make the topping, melt the chocolate in a bowl over hot water, spread it over the cooled caramel layer and leave to cool completely. When cold, cut into small squares.

Gooey Chocolate Fudge Brownies

A good brownie is definitely worth piling into, even at 100 calories per forkful. This is my mother's recipe – these brownies were probably one of the first things I learned to cook. The recipe is blissfully easy and uses only one pan. The resulting brownies are heaven with vanilla ice cream.

Makes 12 brownies

Ingredients

50g chocolate, 70% cocoa
 solids
50g unsalted butter
225g caster sugar

1 egg, beaten
½ teaspoon salt
100g plain flour
vanilla extract

Method

Preheat the oven to 150°C/300°F/Gas 2. Grease a square, 18cm baking tin or 12-hole muffin tin.

Melt the chocolate and butter together in a pan then stir in the remaining ingredients. Pour the mixture into the baking tin or muffin tin and bake for about 15–20 minutes till the top is shiny and the glaze looks slightly cracked.

Jumble Cake

As children we loved this fruit cake as it was fun and not grown up – it had chunks of chocolate and sweet oases of crystallised sugar. It has now become my birthday cake. It travels well, so you will always score 'brownie' or 'cake' points if you take this cake as a present.

Serves 8

Ingredients

175g unsalted butter
100g granulated sugar
3 eggs, beaten
225g self-raising flour
pinch of baking powder

pinch of salt
225g mixed dried fruit
75g chocolate, 70% cocoa
   solids, chopped
75g sugar lumps

Method

Preheat the oven to 160°C/320°F/Gas 1. Line the base and sides of an 8cm deep, 20cm in diameter springform cake tin with baking paper.

Cream the butter and sugar together till pale then add the eggs gradually, beating between each addition.

Next, fold in the flour, baking powder and salt, then fold in the fruit, chocolate and sugar cubes.

Add a little milk if necessary so the mixture just drops off a tablespoon and pour into the prepared cake tin.

Bake for about 30 minutes, till the dome of the cake is just golden brown and a skewer comes out almost clean – remember there is molten chocolate underneath that golden exterior.

Chocolate Beetroot Cake

Don't let the mention of beetroot put you off and don't question how this worthy vegetable packed full of antioxidants sneaked into a chapter glorifying unhealthy eating. The beetroot adds a wonderful richness and sweetness to this gorgeous chocolate cake.

We were filming *The Woman Who Ate Scotland* at a charming farm shop called the Storehouse, just north of Inverness. Owner Fiona MacInnes makes this amazing chocolate beetroot cake which she sells in the shop and at the restaurant. She said people only had to try a sample before they were buying the cakes – and the local raw beetroot sales had also shot up!

I remember it was late on Sunday evening and we had almost finished shooting the episode when Victor, the director, said to me, 'Eat some more chocolate cake. Look like you are really enjoying it.' And I thought, 'I've cracked it, I'm getting paid to eat chocolate cake.'

Fiona uses Green & Black's chocolate beetroot cake recipe with cream cheese icing.

Serves 8

Ingredients

Chocolate Beetroot Cake

100g drinking chocolate
230g self-raising flour
200g caster sugar
100g dark chocolate,
   minimum 70% cocoa solids

125g unsalted butter
250g beetroot, boiled and
   skinned (or buy vacuum-
   packed)
3 large eggs, beaten

Cream Cheese Filling

250g cream cheese
60g unsalted butter, softened

200g icing sugar
icing sugar to dust

Method

Preheat the oven to 180°C/350°F/Gas 4. Grease and line an 18cm round tin.

In a large mixing bowl, sift together the drinking chocolate with the flour, then mix in the sugar. Melt the chocolate and butter together in a bowl over hot water. Purée the cooked beetroot in a food processor, then transfer to a bowl and whisk in the beaten eggs.

Add the beetroot and the chocolate mixtures to the sifted, dry ingredients and beat together thoroughly. Pour the mixture into the cake tin.

Bake in the centre of the oven for 50 minutes or till a skewer inserted in the centre comes out clean. Remove from the oven and leave the cake to stand in its tin for 10 minutes before turning out onto a wire rack to cool. When cooled, cut the cake in half.

To make the icing, beat all the ingredients together till creamy and spread liberally over the bottom half of cake, then sandwich the two halves together and sprinkle icing sugar on top.

Checklist for Foods That Go Against the Nutritional Grain

- Potential weight gain
- Cholesterol elevated levels
- Omega 3 essential fatty acids compromised
- Mood fluctuations
- Lethargy
- Dull skin and lifeless hair
- Disturbed sleep
- Digestive upsets

Ask yourself the question: 'Is what I'm eyeing up to eat really worth it?' If the answer is 'yes' – go for it and enjoy!

Have a Good Healthy Day with a Dinner Party at the End!

Strategy – decide on your treat – and don't write the day off, but eat a balanced diet of protein, complex carbs and fat in small amounts throughout the day.

Breakfast: porridge with yoghurt and nuts and seeds or rye toast and nut butter for sustained slow-release energy.

Snack: apples and some nuts for fibre and protein.

Lunch: veggie soup with an oatcake – fill up on fibre.

Snack: hummus and carrot sticks – more fibre and vitamins.

Evening meal: roasted soya beans, stuffed trout with barley and dates and sticky toffee pudding will all contribute omega 3s to balance some of the saturated fats in the cream for the sticky toffee pudding. There is also fibre in beans, dates and barley to help slow down sugar and protein in beans and trout – so enjoy that pudding!

Exercise: extra! Go for double your usual amount.

Water: drink more if drinking wine and to help your liver process extra toxins.

Bonuses: you are more likely to stick to healthy eating if you know you can have a treat. Occasional treats won't upset your metabolism, so you won't feel deprived and you will continue to stick to the path of good nutrition, won't you?

Index

Note: Recipes are in italic, and listed individually under their title only (and grouped under main subjects and ingredients).